Exercise and Diabetes

Fifth Edition

Hana Abdulaziz Feeney, MS, RD, CSSD
Gwen Hyatt, MS

A special thanks to our course reviewers.

Jeanine Adams, EdD, OTR/L
At-home mom
Haymarket, VA

David Bagby
SimplyFit Fitness Services
Jacksonville, FL

Sarah Emanuel, MS
Manager, Health Promotion
Nebraska Medical Center
Omaha, NE

Troy Huggett, MS
Personal Trainer
Battle Creek, MI

Managing Editor and Text Designer: Karen Thomas
Cover Designer: Rae Anik

ISBN-13: 978-0-9800062-2-3
ISBN-10: 0-9800062-2-8

Unconditional Guarantee
If you are not completely satisfied with the DSWFitness correspondence course *Exercise and Diabetes, 2nd edition,* you may exchange your course or receive a full refund, less shipping and handling charges. Materials must be returned unmarked and intact to our office within 30 days of receiving them. All refunds will be made in the same payment method as received.

Copyright
Copyright 1988, 1996, 2001, 2010, 2011 by Desert Southwest Fitness, Inc. All rights reserved. No part of this work may be reproduced or transmitted in any form or by any means, electronic or mechanical, including photocopying and recording, or by any information storage or retrieval system, except as may be expressly permitted by the 1976 Copyright Act or in writing by the publisher.

Disclaimer
DSWFitness educational products are informational only. The data and information contained in DSWFitness educational products are based upon information from various published as well as unpublished sources and merely represent general training, exercise, and health literature and practices as summarized by the authors and editors. Care has been taken to confirm the accuracy of the information presented and to describe generally accepted practice. However, the author and publisher are not responsible for errors or omissions or for any consequences from application of the information in the educational products. As publisher and distributor of educational products DSWFitness makes no guarantees or warranties, express or implied, regarding the currentness, completeness, or scientific accuracy of this information, nor does the publisher/distributor guarantee or warrant the fitness, marketability, efficacy, or accuracy of this information for any particular purpose. Information from unpublished sources, books, research journals, and articles is not intended to replace the advice or attention of medical or healthcare professionals. This summary is also not intended to direct anyone's behavior or replace anyone's independent professional judgment. If you have a problem with your health, before you embark on any health, fitness, or sports training program, including the programs herein, please seek advice and clearance from a qualified medical or healthcare professional. The publishers have made every effort to trace the copyright holders for borrowed material. If they have inadvertently overlooked any, they will be pleased to make necessary arrangements at the first opportunity.

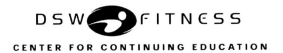

CENTER FOR CONTINUING EDUCATION

602 E. ROGER RD • TUCSON, AZ 85705 • 520.292.0011 • FAX 520.292.0066 • EXAMS@DSWFITNESS.COM • WWW.DSWFITNESS.COM

✳ CONTENTS

1 DIABETES IN THE UNITED STATES   1
Diabetes Mellitus in Racial and Ethnic Groups   2
Diabetes Mellitus in Children   4
Study Questions   5

2 UNDERSTANDING DIABETES MELLITUS   7
Regulation of Blood Glucose   7
Types of Diabetes   8
Symptoms and Complications of Diabetes   13
Social-Psychological Considerations   18
Study Questions   19

3 NUTRITION AND MEDICATIONS FOR DIABETES TREATMENT   21
Nutrition Management   21
Medications   23
Monitoring Blood Glucose   23
Study Questions   26

4 EXERCISE AND DIABETES   27
Guidelines for Diabetes and Exercise   27
Benefits of Exercise   29
Risks of Exercise   30
Contraindications for Exercise   33
Glycemia and Exercise: Know Your Client   33
Study Questions   37

5 EXERCISE DESIGN — 41

Exercise Program Development — 41

Study Questions — 49

6 NUTRITION SURROUNDING EXERCISE — 51

Before Exercise — 51

During Exercise — 52

After Exercise — 52

Treating Hypogylcemia — 53

Hydration — 53

Study Questions — 55

7 SPECIAL CONSIDERATIONS FOR DIABETES AND EXERCISE — 57

Clients Using Insulin — 57

Clients Using Oral Medications and/or Lifestyle Modification — 59

Clients with Gestational Diabetes — 60

Athletes with Diabetes — 61

Older Clients with Diabetes — 64

Group Exercise Considerations — 65

Foot Care for the Physically Active — 66

Study Questions — 68

8 PROFESSIONAL RESPONSIBILITIES — 71

Health Screening for Physical Activity — 71

Monitoring Exercise — 77

Responding to Acute Diabetes Complications — 79

Recordkeeping — 80

Criteria for Termination of Exercise — 81

Contraindications for Exercise — 81

Risk Management — 82

Study Questions — 84

APPENDIX: MONITORING EXERCISE — 85
GLOSSARY — 89
CLIENT HANDOUTS — 91

ANSWER KEYS	117
REFERENCES	125
RESOURCES	129
ABOUT THE AUTHORS	131

1 | DIABETES IN THE UNITED STATES

Diabetes is the sixth leading cause of preventable death in the United States and is a disease that increases the risk of death from the three leading causes of preventable death: heart disease, stroke, and cancer. In 2007, 23.6 million people in the United States had diabetes. Of that number, 5.7 million had not been diagnosed with the condition before being admitted to the hospital for another reason or during a routine office visit (National Institute of Diabetes, Digestive and Kidney Disease [NIDDK] 2009). The estimated lifetime risk for developing diabetes for people born in 2000 is 33% for males and 39% for females (National Institutes of Health [NIH] 2005). Diabetes affects people of all racial and ethnic groups, all ages, and both genders.

There are two primary types of diabetes. Type 2 diabetes mellitus (T2DM) involves the inability of the body to regulate blood glucose levels appropriately due to impaired insulin action and/or secretion. Type 2 diabetes is preventable and is much more prevalent than type 1 diabetes. Type 1 diabetes mellitus (T1DM) involves autoimmune destruction of pancreatic beta cells, resulting in a lack of endogenous insulin production and therefore the inability to regulate blood glucose. At this time, strategies to prevent type 1 diabetes are unknown.

According to the Centers for Disease Control and Prevention (2008b), in addition to those with diagnosed diabetes, many more individuals are at risk for developing type 2 diabetes. The risk of developing type 2 diabetes increases with age. In adults aged 60 years and older, 35.4% are at risk for type 2 diabetes. Seven percent of U.S. adolescents and 25.9% of U.S. adults have impaired fasting glucose (IFG) or prediabetes. IFG prevalence among U.S. adults aged 20 years and older is 21.1% for non-Hispanic blacks, 25.1% for non-Hispanic whites, and 26.1% for Mexican Americans. This data suggest that at least 57 million American adults had prediabetes in 2007.

The costs associated with diabetes are large and increasing. Direct medical costs related to diabetes are $116 billion per year. Average medical expenditures among people with diagnosed diabetes are 2.3 times higher than medical expenditures are for people without the disease. The indirect costs of diabetes, due to disability, work loss, or premature mortality, are $58 billion per year (NIDDK 2009). These costs are disturbing and frustrating considering that type 2 diabetes is preventable. Diabetes is a chronic, costly condition that negatively affects the health and quality of life of millions of individuals, and the rate of the disease is increasing at an alarming rate.

Health experts indicate that the incidence of type 2 diabetes may be related to the following factors: the rise in central body fatness, an increasingly sedentary lifestyle, and a diet of processed foods high in calories. The latest data from the National Center for Health Statistics indicate that 66.3% of U.S. adults, 17% of U.S. adolescents, and 19% of U.S. children are overweight or obese. Eighty-five percent of people with type 2 diabetes are obese (CDC 2008a). As the rates of people being overweight and obese have increased, so has the rate of type 2 diabetes.

Physical activity and a healthy diet help to prevent type 2 diabetes and improve the health and disease management in both type 1 and type 2 diabetes. Achievement and maintenance of a healthy weight and consistent engagement in aerobic exercise help to prevent prediabetes from progressing to type 2 diabetes. Health and fitness professionals have a wonderful opportunity to motivate and guide individuals with diabetes toward better health through exercise.

DIABETES MELLITUS IN RACIAL AND ETHNIC GROUPS

Certain racial and ethnic groups in the U.S. experience diabetes, specifically type 2 diabetes mellitus, more frequently than other groups, possibly due to interactions between genetics; limited access to financial, social, health, and educational resources; language and other logistical barriers; and cultural and socioeconomic status.

Non–Hispanic black individuals and Mexican Americans are 1.8 and 1.7 times, respectively, more likely to have diabetes than non–Hispanic white individuals (NIDDK 2009). Furthermore, American Indian and Alaska Native individuals are 2.2 times more likely to have diabetes than non–Hispanic white individuals (CDC 2007). Interestingly, the rates of diabetes in Native Americans vary by region from 6.0% among Alaska Native adults to 29.3% among American Indian adults in southern Arizona (CDC 2007). Available data indicate that individuals of Asian, Native Hawaiian, and other Pacific Islander ancestry are more than twice as likely as non–Hispanic white individuals to have diagnosed diabetes (NIH 2005). Across racial and ethnic groups, women are more affected by diabetes than men (NIH 2005).

The prevalence of T2DM in every racial and ethnic population is much higher in the United States than in their respective countries of origin. African Americans have been documented to have diabetes up to 10 times more commonly than native African blacks. Mexican Americans living in urban Texas have been shown to have a 65% greater likelihood of having T2DM than Mexicans living in low-income neighborhoods of Mexico City. T2DM affects 54% of male and 37% of female Pima Indians residing in Arizona, compared with 6% of male and 11% of female Pima Indians residing in Mexico (Lee

2003). Pima Indians living in Arizona have one of the highest documented prevalences of diabetes in the world. According to the SEARCH for Diabetes in Youth Study Group, the incidence of T2DM among American Indians aged 15 to 19 years is 49.4%, compared with 5.6% in non-Hispanic whites of the same age group (Writing Group 2007). Pima Indian adolescents in Arizona have the highest reported prevalence of type 2 diabetes mellitus among youth in the United States. Urbanization, which leads to a more sedentary lifestyle and a reliance on processed foods, and dietary changes likely contribute to the increased prevalence of T2DM in these groups.

The diets of many racial and ethnic groups in the United States have significantly less fiber intake and higher consumption of animal fats and processed carbohydrates than traditional Mexican, African, Latin, and Asian diets (Liu, Manson, and Stampfer 2000). A diet that is low in fiber and high in fat and sugar increases the risk for T2DM. The impact of a shift in diet on health is illustrated in studies of Mexican Americans. Those born in the United States are more likely than those born in Mexico to have diets containing more than 30% of calories from fats and less than 25 grams of fiber per day (Dixon, Sundquist, and Winkleby 2000).

Differences in obesity and the effects of obesity on glucose metabolism also have been explored and seem to vary by racial and ethnic group. Genetics also play a role in the development of diabetes and helps to explain racial and ethnic disparities. It is likely there are specific genetic mutations in proteins that regulate glucose metabolism, insulin secretion, and insulin action that vary in different racial and ethnic groups (Abate and Chandalia 2003). Genetic factors seem to modulate the impact of body fat on metabolic pathways that would lead to T2DM (Lee 2003). For example, studies suggest that in individuals of African heritage, beta-cell dysfunction may be the dominant mechanism leading to diabetes in these individuals (Banerji and Lebovitz 1992) whereas insulin resistance appears to be the dominant mechanism leading to T2DM in Caucasian, Asian, and Hispanic people (Lee 2003).

More and more individuals are immigrating to the Unites States. Estimates of what the racial and ethnic composition of the United States population will be in 25 years suggest that more than 50% of the population will include individuals of non-European ancestry, mainly people from Latin America and Asia (Lee 2003). Since acculturation in the United States leads to increased risk of diabetes, racial and ethnic groups should be targeted with culturally sensitive lifestyle interventions that involve exercise to help reduce the risk of developing T2DM.

DIABETES MELLITUS IN CHILDREN

According to the SEARCH for Diabetes in Youth Study Group, the incidence of diabetes mellitus is 24.3% (Writing Group 2007). Among children younger than 10 years of age with the condition, most had type 1 diabetes mellitus, regardless of race and ethnicity. The highest rates of T1DM were observed in non-Hispanic white youth. Overall, the incidence of T2DM among children is still relatively low, with the highest rates among 15- to 19-year-olds from minority groups (Writing Group 2007). Reports indicate that up to 45% of newly diagnosed cases of diabetes among U.S. children and adolescents are classified as T2DM (Neufeld et al. 1998). The prevalence of T2DM among American children is expected to continue to increase and exceed that of T1DM over the next 10 years (Gahagan and Silverstein 2003). This trend will have a major impact on future generations as people diagnosed with diabetes before 40 years of age will experience an average reduction in life expectancy of 12 years for men and 19 years for women (Narayan et al. 2003).

The reason for the increased prevalence of T2DM in children and adolescents is related to many of the same factors that contribute to the development of diabetes in adults. Genes have been identified that are associated with glucose intolerance, insulin resistance, and reduced insulin production (Kempf, Rathmann, and Christian 2008). In addition, environmental factors have been linked to the early onset of diabetes in children and adolescents. These include poor diet, sedentary lifestyle, smoking, and low socio-economic status (Kempf, Rathmann, and Christian 2008). Environmental factors such as these seem to contribute to insulin resistance, impaired beta-cell function, and low-grade chronic inflammation that lead to the development of T2DM.

STUDY QUESTIONS

Complete the following questions. The answer key is on page 117.

1. True or false? Women are disproportionately affected by diabetes compared with men.

2. Describe the lifestyle factors associated with the increased prevalence of diabetes in the US.

3. What ethnic groups experience higher rates of diabetes compared to non-Hispanics whites (Caucasians)?

4. Which is more prevalent in children and adolescents, type 1 or type 2 diabetes?

5. What environmental factors increase the risk of type 2 diabetes in children and adolescents?

6. True or false? Central body fat is associated with an increased incidence of type 2 diabetes.

2 | UNDERSTANDING DIABETES MELLITUS

If you are a veteran of the fitness industry or are just beginning your career as a fitness professional, at some point you will encounter a personal training client or a student in your group exercise class who has diabetes. It is also likely that you will encounter clients who are unaware they have diabetes or have trouble controlling their diabetes. Diabetes is classified as a metabolic disorder characterized by high levels of blood glucose resulting from defects in insulin secretion, insulin action, or both. The four types of diabetes mellitus are: type 1 diabetes mellitus (T1DM), type 2 diabetes mellitus (T2DM), gestational diabetes mellitus (GDM), and latent autoimmune diabetes of the adult (LADA). Each form shares some defect related to insulin. T1DM relates to the absence of endogenous insulin due to immune destruction of beta cells. T2DM involves the inability of the body to appropriately regulate blood glucose levels due to impaired insulin action and/or secretion. It is preventable and is much more prevalent than T1DM. GDM occurs during pregnancy secondary to insulin resistance. Insulin resistance is the impaired action of insulin. LADA is similar to T1DM and develops slowly in adults.

REGULATION OF BLOOD GLUCOSE

Glucose is the fuel most readily available for use by muscle cells, and it is the only fuel available to the brain and the nervous system. It is the body's main energy source and is utilized in every cell of the body. Insulin is an essential hormone that regulates glucose, fat, and protein metabolism and affects the way the body uses food for fuel. When insulin does not work properly or when there is insufficient production of insulin, blood glucose levels remain high. Hyperglycemia (high blood glucose level) is quite damaging and leads to the long-term complications of diabetes, which include neuropathy, retinopathy, nephropathy, and atherosclerosis. A diagnosis of diabetes occurs when fasting blood glucose is above normal (>126 mg/dl) on two separate occasions (American Diabetes Association 2008).

Glucose is formed exogenously (externally) from food or endogenously (internally) in the liver and muscles. Following a meal, the carbohydrate in food is broken down into glucose by stomach acid and digestive enzymes. As carbohydrate is metabolized, glucose moves from the gastrointestinal tract into the bloodstream. Glucose must then move

7

from the bloodstream into cells to be used as energy. The liver and muscles store glucose in the form of glycogen.

The movement of glucose out of the blood into a cell requires the hormone insulin. Insulin is released by the pancreas to enable the body to metabolize glucose. Under normal physiological conditions, insulin is released from the pancreas in precise amounts relative to the rise in blood glucose and binds to a cell receptor. This binding signals the walls of cells to open and take in the circulating blood glucose. As glucose is absorbed and metabolized by the cells, the level of circulating blood glucose drops so that blood glucose levels remain relatively stable. The only time insulin is not required to move glucose from the blood and into the cells is during and immediately following exercise. When insulin levels rise, endogenous production of glucose slows. Therefore, insulin has two main functions:

1. It allows glucose, from food or internal production, to pass into cells out of the bloodstream and to be used for energy.
2. It assists in shutting off excess internal glucose production in the liver and muscles.

When additional glucose is needed beyond what is provided from food, endogenous glucose production occurs. Glycogen is broken down into glucose and released in small amounts from the liver to keep blood glucose levels stable or is released in larger amounts from the muscle to fuel exercise.

TYPES OF DIABETES

The four types of diabetes each have different etiologies and risk factors. The primary treatment goal for all four types is to regulate blood glucose level.

Type 1 Diabetes Mellitus (T1DM)

Type 1 diabetes mellitus usually develops in children or young adults but can occur at any age. Only 5% to 10% of all diabetics are type 1, or insulin-dependent (Bellenir 1999). The risk of developing T1DM is higher than virtually all other severe chronic diseases of childhood. Peak incidence occurs during puberty, around 10 to 12 years of age in girls and 12 to 14 years of age in boys. However, the onset of T1DM is not limited to childhood; the condition can develop later in life, most often before 30 years of age.

Type 1 diabetes mellitus: etiology. Type 1 diabetes is an autoimmune disease. Autoimmunity in T1DM results in the immune system attacking and destroying the insulin-producing beta cells of the pancreas. Without properly functioning beta cells, the pancreas cannot produce a significant amount of insulin, and this leads to an elevation of blood glucose levels.

Although researchers do not know exactly what causes the body's immune system to attack the beta cells, two reasons seem to be linked to T1DM autoimmunity: heredity and environmental factors (including viral or chemical agents). Strategies to prevent T1DM are unknown; however, inflammation in the pancreas and inflammatory markers have been identified prior to the destruction of beta cells, indicating a possibility of identifying high-risk patients for intervention.

Type 1 diabetes mellitus: symptoms. Individuals with T1DM need an external source of insulin from injections or an infusion pump to survive. The deficiency of insulin rapidly leads to hyperglycemia if not treated. Glucose that remains in the bloodstream will overflow and be cleared through the kidneys into the urine. Increased urine production may cause the body to become quickly dehydrated.

Individuals with T1DM have the propensity to develop ketoacidosis. Without insulin, the body begins to burn fat and protein for energy because it is unable to utilize glucose. The byproduct of fat and protein metabolism is ketones. As ketones in the blood begin to rise, the blood becomes more acidic, leading to a condition called ketoacidosis. This condition causes the individual to become very ill with symptoms that include abdominal pain, severe nausea, vomiting, rapid breathing, and possibly diabetic coma.

Early symptoms of type 1 diabetes include:

- Frequent urination
- Excessive thirst
- Excessive fatigue
- Sudden weight loss
- Constant or extreme hunger
- Blurred vision
- Repeated or hard-to-heal infections of the skin
- Increased gum or urinary tract infections
- Dry, itchy skin
- Tingling or loss of feeling in the hands or feet

Symptoms in children can often mimic the flu; however, they will be constant and increase in severity until T1DM is diagnosed.

Type 1 Diabetes Mellitus: treatment. The first goal of T1DM treatment is to avoid extreme blood glucose fluctuations. Type 1 diabetes mellitus is a life-long condition and exogenous insulin must be administered daily. People with T1DM require exogenous insulin via injection or continuous insulin infusion pump. The goal in managing T1DM is to adequately provide insulin to normalize blood glucose levels, prevent hypoglycemia (low blood glucose level), and to lessen the effects of long-term complications of the condition. Treatment requires a regimen that typically includes self-glucose monitoring several times a day and insulin administration throughout the day to achieve as-close-to-normal glucose control as possible while avoiding hypoglycemia. A very significant risk from exogenous insulin use is hypoglycemia. Hypoglycemia is the most dangerous complication of type 1 diabetes, or any diabetes managed with insulin, as hypoglycemia can result in coma or death very quickly. A carefully planned diet and regular participation in physical activity optimizes blood glucose control and helps to prevent the complications of diabetes. Your clients with T1DM should be working with a team of diabetes professionals that include a physician, certified diabetes educator, and a registered dietitian. The fitness professional also plays a role on this team.

Type 1.5 or LADA (Adult Slow Onset Diabetes)

Latent autoimmune diabetes of the adult (LADA) is a form of diabetes similar to T1DM that develops slowly in adults and has become increasingly prevalent in the U.S. population. As with T1DM, LADA is an autoimmune condition that leads to the destruction of pancreatic beta cells, resulting in the inability to produce insulin. Exogenous insulin is the primary treatment for LADA, as it is for T1DM. Typically, T1DM develops in childhood or adolescence; however, many cases of T1DM are now diagnosed in adults, and this is a new trend (Colberg 2009). LADA differs from T1DM in the way that the disease progresses. LADA progresses slowly and T1DM progresses very quickly. For example, when an individual is diagnosed with T1DM, he or she will present with significant hyperglycemia and ketoacidosis. In LADA, the progression of the disease is slow and control of blood glucose can be achieved with diet, exercise, and/or oral medications for a period of months. This is not possible with a classic case of T1DM. However, lifestyle changes and oral medications will not adequately control blood glucose in the long-term, and individuals with LADA are eventually placed on insulin. Often, people in the beginning stages of LADA are misdiagnosed with T2DM because their body is making some insulin but not enough to adequately control blood glucose. Up to 20% of people diagnosed with T2DM actually have LADA (Colberg 2009). The progression to insulin is much quicker than it is for an individual with T2DM. Additionally, insulin resistance is not a component of LADA.

Type 2 Diabetes Mellitus (T2DM)

Type 2 diabetes is more common than type 1 and accounts for approximately 90% to 95% of Americans diagnosed with the condition. Of these, approximately one-third are unaware they have the disease until they are diagnosed as a result of a hospital or office visit for another reason. The risk for T2DM increases with age; however, T2DM in children and adolescents has become increasingly common. The American Heart Association (2009) names T2DM a one of the major modifiable risk factors for heart disease and stroke (along with cigarette smoking, high blood pressure, high cholesterol, obesity, and lack of exercise).

Type 2 diabetes mellitus: etiology. Major predisposing risk factors for T2DM are obesity, family history, sedentary lifestyle, and advanced age. According to the American Diabetes Association (2008), nearly 18.4% of the U.S. population between 65 and 74 years of age has the disease, and 80% of people diagnosed with the disease are considered to be obese. People who are not obese but who are sedentary are also at increased risk for T2DM. It has been noted that T2DM is more likely to occur in obese individuals who carry excess fat around their abdomen with greater amounts of visceral fat (fat within the abdominal cavity). These individuals are referred to as having central obesity, or an upper-body fat distribution pattern.

Two mechanisms lead to the development of T2DM: (1) a defect occurs in the beta cells where there is an impaired capacity for insulin secretion and (2) a reduction in insulin sensitivity. Reduced insulin sensitivity results in a diminished ability to use insulin because it can no longer bind to the insulin receptor sites on cell surfaces or cells lack sufficient insulin receptors. Excess body fat appears to enhance insulin resistance and negatively impact pancreatic beta-cell insulin secretion. It is important to remember that some individuals with T2DM may be severely insulin-resistant despite a minimal accumulation of body fat. Body-fat cells secrete proinflammatory compounds that contribute to chronic inflammation, and low-grade inflammation contributes to reduced insulin secretion and to insulin resistance.

People with T2DM either have significantly impaired insulin secretion and require insulin for glycemic control or still produce some insulin and rely on oral medications and lifestyle modifications to manage their blood glucose levels. As the disease progresses, more of the pancreatic beta cells die off, and the dependence on insulin increases.

With inadequate insulin or with insulin resistance, cells fail to get the glucose they need. Therefore, blood glucose increases. In the early stages of T2DM, insulin production increases to compensate for insulin resistance. Without intervention, hyperglycemia progresses and, as with T1DM, the kidneys are unable to reabsorb the excess glucose, and it passes some of the glucose into the urine.

Type 2 Diabetes Mellitus: Risk Factors

- Sedentary lifestyle
- Family history of type 2 diabetes
- Ethnicity (African American, Hispanic and Latino, American Indian, Asian American)
- History of gestational diabetes
- High blood pressure
- Low HDL cholesterol and high triglycerides
- Excess abdominal body fat
- Polycystic ovarian syndrome
- History of heart disease

(ADA 2008)

Type 2 diabetes mellitus: symptoms. Early symptoms of T2DM include:

- Increased thirst, especially at night
- Increased urination, especially at night
- Fatigue
- Blurred vision
- Slow healing of the skin
- Gum and urinary tract infections

Type 2 diabetes mellitus: treatment. Exercise and dietary change may be enough to reverse T2DM by improving insulin resistance. Participation in moderate exercise (30 minutes on most days of the week) has been shown to reduce the progression of impaired glucose tolerance to T2DM (Tuomilheto et al. 2001). The use of oral medications to increase endogenous insulin production and/or insulin sensitivity also helps to manage blood glucose when diet and exercise are not sufficient. When lifestyle changes and oral medications do not adequately prevent hyperglycemia, it becomes necessary to include exogenous insulin to improve blood glucose control. Approximately 40% of people with type 2 diabetes require insulin injections (Bellenir 1999).

Gestational Diabetes (GDM)

When diabetes occurs during pregnancy it is termed gestational diabetes. Gestational diabetes is usually temporary; however, it increases the lifetime risk for T2DM. It is most often discovered when a woman has a urine test or a routine blood test for glucose during a visit to her physician during pregnancy. Once GDM is diagnosed, the woman may or may not require insulin. Her blood sugar will need to be monitored closely during the pregnancy. Exercise is encouraged for those with GDM to improve both maternal and fetal health.

Gestational diabetes: etiology. Pregnancy is a time of significant increase in insulin resistance. The body needs more insulin during pregnancy as hormones produced by the placenta oppose the action of insulin, making insulin less effective. When the pancreas is unable to meet this increased need for insulin, hyperglycemia occurs. Insulin requirements tend to drop in the first trimester and increase in the second and third trimester. The result is high blood glucose levels beginning the 24th to 26th week of pregnancy, which is when women are tested for GDM.

The risk factors for gestational diabetes are (Dornhorst and Rossi 1998; Mattola 2008):

- Sedentary lifestyle
- Family history of diabetes in a first-degree relative
- Overweight or obesity prior to pregnancy
- Over the age of 35

- Prior deliveries of large-birthweight babies (over 10 lb)
- Repeated miscarriages or spontaneous abortions in previous pregnancies
- A history of glucose in the urine in a previous or current pregnancy
- A history of GDM
- Family history of diabetes
- Ethnicity (Hispanic, South Asian, Asian, or African descent)

Gestational diabetes: treatment. The American Diabetes Association recommends that all pregnant women be tested for diabetes between the 24th and 26th weeks of pregnancy. Often, treatment with a carefully monitored food plan and consistent exercise is enough to control blood glucose. Recommendations for exercise, weight gain, and energy and nutrient intake are similar for pregnant women whose pregnancies are not complicated by GDM. When diet and exercise do not adequately control glycemia, insulin is required. Most oral hypoglycemic agents are contraindicated during pregnancy; however, glyburide may be used.

Exercise is necessary for a healthy pregnancy. Regular exercise prior to pregnancy reduces the risk of GDM (Zhang et al. 2006). Exercise is also a safe and viable option for managing blood glucose during pregnancy.

After delivery, blood glucose levels usually return to normal; however, gestational diabetes increases a woman's risk for having diabetes later. Up to 60% of women who develop GDM will develop T2DM within four years after delivery (Kelly and Booth 2004) and multiple pregnancies with GDM increases the risk even more.

SYMPTOMS AND COMPLICATIONS OF DIABETES

Type 1 diabetes is frequently diagnosed in children and young adults. Early symptoms appear suddenly. Type 2 diabetes usually occurs after the age of 40 but is increasingly developing in children and adolescents. It has been diagnosed in children as young as the age of 8. Unlike the symptoms of T1DM, the symptoms of T2DM appear gradually. Symptoms of undiagnosed diabetes include the following:

- Frequent urination, especially at night
- Abnormal thirst
- Constant/extreme hunger
- Rapid loss of weight (generally in T1DM)
- Excessive fatigue
- Irritability, weakness, fatigue
- Blurred vision
- Increased infections of gums, urinary tract, eyes, skin
- Dry, itchy skin, slow-healing skin infections
- Tingling or loss of feeling in hands or feet

In T1DM, insufficient insulin that leads to hyperglycemia may progress to ketoacidosis, which is when a diagnosis of T1DM often occurs. Once diagnosed, it is important to provide adequate insulin to prevent ketoacidosis. Ketoacidosis does not occur in T2DM. Symptoms of ketoacidosis include:

- Dehydration, stomach pain
- Nausea
- Fruity breath
- Drowsiness, vomiting
- Rapid breathing
- Headache
- Muscle pain

Fatigue, increased urination, and thirst are the most common and pronounced symptoms of both type 1 and type 2 diabetes. Because cells have difficulty metabolizing glucose for energy, muscle fatigue occurs quickly. The excess fluid needed to process the overflow of glucose in the kidneys causes frequent urination. Frequent urination results in water loss and increases thirst and dehydration. These symptoms are often what lead to a diagnosis of diabetes and are symptoms of uncontrolled diabetes.

Short-Term Complications Of Diabetes

In the short-term, hypoglycemia (low blood glucose) is the most dangerous complication for people on insulin or taking an oral hypoglycemic agent that increases insulin production. The symptoms of hypoglycemia include:

- Cold or clammy skin
- Buzzing in ears
- Dizziness or lightheadedness
- Double or blurred vision
- Elevated heart rate
- Inability to do basic math
- Insomnia
- Irritability
- Confusion
- Paleness
- Shaking hands
- Extreme fatigue
- Headache
- Nausea
- Nervousness
- Nightmares
- Poor coordination

- Restlessness
- Slurred speech
- Sweating
- Visual spots
- Extreme hunger; panicky hunger
- Loss of consciousness
- Seizures
- Coma

Ketoacidosis

Diabetic ketoacidosis (DKA) is a life-threatening complication of diabetes that occurs in the short-term due to near complete deficiency of insulin. DKA occurs most often in T1DM due to the reliance on insulin to control glucose. Often when an individual is diagnosed with T1DM they will present with DKA. DKA can occur in any individual with known diabetes who fails to take adequate insulin and/or control hyperglycemia. DKA does not generally affect those with T2DM; however, during periods of significant physiological stress, such as during an infection or wound healing, DKA can occur in uncontrolled T2DM. Symptoms of DKA are:

- Sluggishness
- Extreme fatigue
- Extreme thirst, despite large fluid intake
- Dry mouth, swollen tounge
- Constant urination
- Vomiting, nausea
- Fruity smell to breath or sweat, similar to nail polish remover (acetone)
- Hyperventilation, at first rapid and shallow, then progressively deeper and less rapid
- Aggression
- Extreme weight loss; muscle wasting
- Yeast infections

The symptoms of DKA develop over days or weeks. However, fatigue, thirst, increased urination, nausea, fruity smell to breath, sweat, and hyperventilation can be present in your exercisng clients experiencing ketoacidosis due to hyperglycemia and inadequate insulin. It is important to watch for these symptoms because they can rapidly progress to more signicant problems, such as loss of consciousness or coma. Monitor blood glucose level and stop exercise when needed. If hyperglycemia is identified and if ketoacidosis is suspected, encourage your client to check his or her urine for ketones, administer insulin appropriately, and have the client rest and drink fluids.

Long-Term Complications Of Diabetes

The following complications affect people with type 1 and type 2 diabetes mellitus. It is unlikely that these complications would develop during GDM due to its short duration. If hyperglycemia continued into the postpartum period, T2DM may be diagnosed. Very rarely is T1DM a complication of GDM. Unfortunately, many people first become aware that they have diabetes when they develop a life-threatening, long-term complication of the disease, meaning that they have unknowingly had T2DM for quite a long time. Long-term complications associated with diabetes include cardiovascular disease, autonomic and peripheral neuropathy (nerve damage), renal (kidney) disease, peripheral ulcerations, and autonomic nervous system dysfunction.

According to the National Institute of Diabetes, Digestive and Kidney Diseases (2009), the most common complications of long-term diabetes include cardiovascular disease, blindness, nephropathy, neuropathy and amputations, dental disease, and prenatal complications.

Cardiovascular disease. Hyperglycemia negatively affects the artery walls and may be involved in the initial development of atherosclerosis. Hyperglycemia contributes to damage of the intima, the innermost lining of vessel walls. Abnormalities of vessel wall structure and function can result in several health-related problems such as transient ischemic attack (TIA), which causes a brief interruption of blood flow to the brain and atherosclerosis. Angina pectoris, heart attack, and peripheral vascular disease are other disorders common in diabetes. In 2004, heart disease and stroke contributed to the death of 84% of people aged 65 and older with diabetes. The risks of heart disease and stroke are two to four times higher for adults with diabetes than it is for adults without the disease. Hypertension is present in 75% of people with diabetes. It has also been demonstrated that hyperglycemia increases very low-density lipoprotein (VLDL), the precursor to low-density lipoprotein (LDL) cholesterol particles. Hyperglycemia is also associated with increases in triglycerides and c-reactive protein (CRP).

Blindness. Diabetes increases the risk of retinopathy and blindness. It is the leading cause of new cases of blindness in adults, causing 12,000 to 24,000 new cases of blindness annually.

Nephropathy. In 2005, 44% of new cases of kidney failure were caused by diabetes. People who initiated dialysis as treatment for end-stage kidney failure numbered 46,739, and 178,689 people with end-stage kidney disease due to diabetes were living on dialysis or with a kidney transplant.

Neuropathy and amputations. Hyperglycemia results in the progressive loss of the protective insulation that surrounds nerves. Tingling and burning of the feet are among the first signs of damage of the sensory nerves. These sensations may be followed by pain and discomfort in the lower extremities, especially at night. Numbness can occur, making it hard to feel cuts, blisters, or hot spots on the feet. Neuropathy can lead to impairment of peripheral vascular circulation and the development of peripheral vascular disease (PVD). Mild to severe nerve damage occurs in 60% to 70% of people with diabetes. Clients with PVD are also at increased risk of cardiovascular disease. Signs of PVD include pain in the calves when walking, alopecia (hair loss), cold feet, weak or no pulse in feet, numbness and tingling, weak legs, burning or aching in the feet or toes, slow-healing leg and foot abrasions, and discoloration in the legs leading down to the toes.

Nearly one-third of adults with diabetes lose sensation in the feet. Fitness professionals need to be aware of this when working with clients with diabetes. Due to severe nerve damage in the extremities, the majority of nontraumatic amputations occur in people with diabetes. Lower-limb amputations were performed on 71,000 people with diabetes in 2004.

Dental disease. People with diabetes have two times the risk of periodontal disease than people without diabetes. When diabetes is not controlled, the risk is tripled.

Prenatal complications. Birth defects and miscarriage are risks to women with diabetes. Hyperglycemia prior to conception and during the first trimester can cause birth defects in 5% to 10% of pregnancies and miscarriage in 15% to 20% of pregnancies. Hyperglycemia during the second and third trimester increases the birth weight of babies.

Prevention of Long-Term Diabetes Complications

The long-term complications of diabetes have a significant impact on the morbidity, mortality, and quality of life of people with diabetes. Fortunately, with the help of loved ones and healthcare practitioners, people with diabetes can take control of their health and work toward the prevention of diabetes complications.

Glucose control helps to prevent hyperglycemia. Long-term trials have indicated that every percentage point drop in hemoglobin A1C (blood test) can reduce the risk of microvascular complications (eye, kidney, and nerve disease) by 40% (NIDDK 2009). Exercise plays an integral role in managing blood glucose, in addition to blood pressure. Blood pressure control reduces the risk of cardiovascular disease among people with diabetes by 33% to 50% and the microvascular complications by about 33%. For every 10 mmHg reduction in systolic blood pressure, the risk for diabetes-related complications is reduced by 12% (NIDDK 2009). The decline in kidney function can be reduced by 30% to 70% by detecting and treating kidney disease early and by lowering blood pressure (NIDDK 2009). Blood pressure is often treated with angiotensin-converting enzyme (ACE) inhibitors and angiotensin receptor blockers (ARBs) as they have a dual effect in protecting kidney function and reducing blood pressure. Be sure to be aware of the medications that your clients are taking to prevent the long-term complications of diabetes. Exercise also contributes to lipid control, which may reduce the risk of cardiovascular complications by 20% to 50% (NIDDK 2009).

SOCIAL-PSYCHOLOGICAL CONSIDERATIONS

Many social-psychological problems, both interpersonal and financial, can arise as a result of a chronic illness such as diabetes. The condition itself makes daily life more difficult. Special attention must be given to nutritional requirements, and in many cases medication requirements, to manage the disease. Constant monitoring and injections are required for a person with type 1 diabetes.

Depression, decreased self-esteem, and worry are not uncommon in people with diabetes. The disease can affect the entire family and social network. It is important to know when to refer someone to an appropriate healthcare provider. If you are ever in doubt about a client's symptoms or psychological or physical status, refer him or her to a healthcare provider right away.

STUDY QUESTIONS

Complete the following questions. The answer key is on pages 117–119.

1. Describe how glucose is produced.

2. What are the primary functions of insulin?

3. True or false? The onset of type 1 diabetes is always in childhood.

4. Describe the differences between the pathophysiology of type 1 and type 2 diabetes.

5. What are the early symptoms of diabetes?

6. List five risk factors for gestational diabetes.

7. Describe the symptoms of ketoacidosis. In which type of diabetes, type 1, type 2 or gestational, is there a risk for this condition?

8. Describe the symptoms of hypoglycemia.

9. What are the long-term complications of diabetes?

10. For every 1% drop in the hemoglobin A1C the risk of long-term complications is reduced by _____.

3 | NUTRITION AND MEDICATIONS FOR DIABETES TREATMENT

Type 1 diabetes mellitus cannot be cured, but it can be managed. Type 2 diabetes mellitus can be "cured," meaning that blood glucose levels can return to normal with proper treatment. However, the individual will forever be at increased risk for high blood glucose levels. Controlling diabetes means keeping blood glucose ranges close to normal as much of the time as possible. Because diabetes is a disease in which the body has difficulty using food, proper nutritional management is a cornerstone of treatment. Diet, exercise, medication, and blood glucose monitoring are essential to the optimal management of glycemia. Excess body fat, smoking, stress, and illness adversely impact the disease. The best way to achieve a balance of all these factors is to work with a team of qualified healthcare professionals, which may include a doctor, registered dietitian, diabetic educator, nurse, and exercise specialist.

NUTRITION MANAGEMENT

The first and major goal of nutrition management for diabetes is to maintain a normal glucose level. This is accomplished by establishing an appropriate meal plan. Meal planning involves providing adequate nutrients and the appropriate number of calories to maintain a desirable body weight, glucose level, and lipid profile. The amount of physical activity in which the individual participates and medication also figure into the food management plan.

The American Dietetic Association has the following goals for guiding individuals with diabetes (Franz et al. 2008):

- Achieve and maintain blood glucose levels in the normal range or as close to normal as safely possible.
- Achieve and maintain a lipid and lipoprotein profile that reduces the risk for vascular disease.
- Achieve and maintain blood pressure levels of less than 120/80 mmHg or as close to normal as safely possible.
- Prevent or delay the development of chronic complications associated with diabetes by modifying nutrient intake and lifestyle.

Chapter Three

- Address nutrition needs, taking into account personal and cultural preferences and willingness to change.
- Maintain the pleasure of eating by only limiting food choices when indicated by scientific evidence.
- For individuals treated with insulin or oral medications that stimulate insulin production, provide self-management training for safe conduct of exercise, including the prevention and treatment of hypoglycemia, and diabetes treatment during acute illness.

Carbohydrate (CHO) is the body's main source of energy. Nutrient-dense dietary sources of CHO include fruit, milk, cereals, whole-grain foods, intact whole grains, legumes, and starchy vegetables. These foods contain valuable antioxidants and fiber to protect against disease. Antioxidants are found in all plant foods and protect the body against the long-term effects of hyperglycemia. Fiber is found in whole-grain foods (breads, pasta, crackers) and whole grains (oats, barley, rice), fruits, vegetables, nuts, and legumes. Fiber gives structure to some foods. It cannot be digested by the body and so has no calories and will not increase blood glucose levels. Fiber increases the sensation of fullness and thus assists with calorie control. Fiber helps to maintain optimal glucose ranges by promoting calorie control and absorbing glucose. High-fiber diets are associated with better glycemic control and weight management.

Others sources of CHO in the diet include added sugars that lack nutrients and are calorie-dense. Added sugars are found in soda, juice, condiments, cereals, breads, crackers, candy, desserts, baked goods, and many other foods. These foods should be avoided.

When digested, CHO increases blood glucose. The more CHO consumed, the greater blood glucose levels increase. Fiber, fat, and protein slow digestion, and, therefore, slow the rate at which blood glucose levels increase. Fiber slows the absorption of food, which helps to keep the levels of glucose and insulin steady. Fiber, particularly soluble fiber, absorbs glucose in the digestive tract and prevents the blood glucose level from surging. Increased amounts of dietary fiber is associated with lower blood glucose levels overall. Fat and protein also slow digestion and cause blood glucose levels to increase more slowly when consumed with carbohydrate. However, certain types of protein and fat-rich foods also negatively affect insulin action. Therefore, careful attention must be paid to both the type and amount of protein and fat in the diet. Lipid management is important because of the relationship between blood lipids and diabetes and heart disease.

The main determinant of blood glucose levels following a meal is the amount of CHO consumed. It is best for the CHO to be consumed in an unprocessed, nutrient-dense form and to be balanced with healthy protein and fat-rich foods. Consumption of smaller amounts of CHO spread throughout the day allows an individual to maintain better blood glucose control compared with large amounts of CHO consumed in one meal or snack.

Proper management of calories and meal planning, combined with exercise, results in realistic weight management. Maintaining a desirable body weight is an important factor in controlling diabetes and may even lead to a reduction or elimination of medication for people with T2DM or GDM.

Many approaches to meal planning are available to individuals with diabetes. Nutrient awareness, portion control, and food choices are all part of successful meal planning. An individual with diabetes should consult with a registered dietitian who has experience working with clients with diabetes to develop an individualized meal-planning approach. To find a registered dietitian for your client, visit the American Dietetics Association website at www.eatright.org. With careful education and guidance from healthcare providers it is possible to make meal planning more flexible and enjoyable, while at the same time controlling blood glucose and lipid levels.

MEDICATIONS

The two major classifications of medications used in the treatment of diabetes are insulin and oral hypoglycemic agents. Information detailing the six classes of oral agents and insulin can be found in chapter 8.

Insulin is always used in the treatment of T1DM and can be used for the treatment of T2DM. Insulin is injected or infused subcutaneously via a pump. Insulin injection or infusion allows for an increase in the amount of insulin in the body to facilitate activation and binding with receptors on cell surfaces to allow glucose to enter the cells. With inadequate insulin, hyperglycemia occurs. When excess amounts of insulin are administered, hypoglycemia occurs, which can become an acutely emergent situation.

Oral hypoglycemic agents can be used by themselves, in combination with each other, or with insulin. Each class of hypoglycemic agent has a unique mechanism for lowering blood glucose levels. Hypoglycemia is less of a concern with oral agents than it is with insulin. However, hypoglycemia can occur if the medication increases insulin output by the pancreas. Medications that increase insulin production are sulfonylureas and metglinitizides.

Questions you and your client have about medications, proper injection sites, or alterations in dosage should be directed to the client's physician or healthcare provider.

MONITORING BLOOD GLUCOSE

To prevent the complications associated with diabetes, your client must know how to measure and monitor his or her blood glucose levels, or blood sugar level. Testing blood sugar is the only way to know whether the blood sugar level is too high, too low, or just right. Testing allows your client to recognize if his or her treatment is effective and to avoid the acute complication of hypoglycemia.

Two different tests for measuring blood sugar are:

1. Self-monitoring of blood glucose (SMBG)
2. Hemoglobin A1C test

Together, these tests allow your client to get a complete picture of his or her blood sugar status.

Self-Monitoring of Blood Glucose (SMBG)

Self-monitoring of blood glucose (SMBG) involves a finger-stick test that is done using a blood-glucose meter to check the current blood sugar level. SMBG tells your clients what their blood sugar is at the time of the test.

SMBG using a blood glucose meter helps to see how food, physical activity, and medication affect blood sugar. Because many factors affect blood glucose levels, it is important to regularly monitor blood sugar levels, particularly surrounding exercise. The information obtained from regular SMBG will allow your clients to successfully manage their blood glucose levels day-by-day or even hour-by-hour. Encourage your clients to keep a record of their test results to review with their healthcare providers.

Normal blood glucose levels are controlled tightly by the body to stay between 70 and 120 mg/dl. The American Academy of Clinical Endocrinologists (2008) recommends that most people with diabetes aim for the following SMBG goals:

Before meals	70–110 mg/dl
2 hours after meals	<140 mg/dl
At bedtime	100–140 mg/dl

The American Diabetes Association (2008) recommends the following goals:

Before meals	70–130 mg/dl
1–2 hours after meals	<180 mg/dl

Your clients' blood sugar goals may be different from these ideal goals. Ask clients to establish goals with their healthcare provider and to share those goals with you. Your clients may have specific blood glucose goals surrounding exercise.

Hemoglobin A1C Test

The hemoglobin A1C test is a simple lab test that shows the average amount of sugar that has been in the blood over the last three months. The healthcare provider does the test by taking a small sample of blood and sending it to a lab. The hemoglobin A1C test shows if, on average, a person's blood sugar is close to normal or too high. It is the best test to tell if blood sugar is under control. Health practitioners should describe hemoglobin A1C test results as "average blood glucose."

The hemoglobin A1C goal for people with diabetes is less than 6.5% or average blood glucose level less than 150 mg/dl on average (see the chart on page 25). A change in the treatment plan is almost always needed if the test result is over 8% or average 205 mg/dl.

A1C and Estimated Ave Glucose

A1C %	3-Month Ave Blood Sugar
4.0	65
4.5	83
5.0	100
5.5	118
6.0	135
6.5	153
7.0	170
7.5	187
8.0	204
8.5	222
9.0	240
9.5	258
10.0	275
10.5	293
11.0	310
11.5	328
12.0	345

A new way to understand how well your client is managing his or her diabetes.

(Adapted from American Diabetes Association.)

Continuous Glucose Monitor

Each year new technology is available to improve the quality of life and health of people with diabetes. An important new technology to consider for active individuals with diabetes is a continuous glucose monitoring system (CGMS). CGMS is an FDA-approved device that records blood sugar levels throughout the day and night. A tiny glucose-sensing device called a sensor is inserted just under the skin of the abdomen. The sensor measures the level of glucose in the interstitial fluids every 10 seconds and sends the information wirelessly to a monitor that attaches to a belt or the waistline of pants. CGMS does not eliminate the need for SMBG. Results of at least four finger stick blood sugar readings are taken with a standard glucose meter and entered into the monitor for calibration throughout the day.

The continuous glucose monitor is intended to discover trends in glucose levels, which is crucial surrounding exercise. The continuous glucose monitor enables individuals with diabetes to take early action to prevent the occurrence or severity of a hypo- or hyperglycemic reaction to exercise. Appropriate adjustments in your client's treatment plan will be made when using the CGMS.

STUDY QUESTIONS

Complete the following questions. The answer key is on page 119.

1. What healthcare professionals may be managing your clients' health and included on the healthcare team?

2. What is the first goal of the nutritional management of diabetes?

3. What type of diet is associated with a lower risk of diabetes and improved glycemic control?

4. True or false? Oral medications can be used by both type 1 and type 2 diabetes clients.

5. What is considered "normal" blood glucose?

6. True or false? Only people with type 1 diabetes have to self-monitor their blood glucose levels.

4 | EXERCISE AND DIABETES

Exercise is an important component of diabetes treatment. A regular exercise program enhances the body's ability to maintain healthy blood glucose control by increasing glucose utilization and by increasing insulin sensitivity. Exercise results in an increase in the affinity for and the number of insulin receptors on cell surfaces. Existing receptors work better, perhaps by binding the insulin more tightly. Remember, receptors assist in the passage of insulin out of the bloodstream and into the cell, thus reducing the amount of circulating glucose and the need for medication.

GUIDELINES FOR DIABETES AND EXERCISE

Diabetes is not a reason to avoid exercise. Exercise for the individual with diabetes is important whether it is performed in a medically based setting, in a community-based group-exercise program, with a personal trainer, or individually at home. Sometimes, general exercise guidelines are not sufficient when working with a client who has diabetes. It is important that each individual client become familiar with his or her specific blood glucose pattern in relation to physical activity. Based on daily blood sugar curves, the client and his or her healthcare provider and exercise practitioner can appropriately design an exercise program and strategy.

For the client with diabetes to enjoy physical activity safely, certain precautions must be taken. The following are exercise guidelines and considerations for working with people who have diabetes.

- Obtain a medical release from the client's physician or healthcare provider prior to beginning or modifying an exercise program.
- Ensure that your client checks his or her blood glucose level prior to engaging in exercise. Do not initiate exercise if blood glucose levels are less than 100 mg/dl or greater than 250 mg/dl with ketones or blood glucose levels are greater than 300 mg/dl without ketones. In addition, the physician should establish the participant's acceptable blood glucose upper limit allowable for exercise.
- It is important to begin your client at entry exercise levels and progress the client gradually in his or her exercise program. Clients should in-

crease only one exercise variable of their exercise program during any given workout session. Exercise variables include frequency, duration, resistance, and number of repetitions or sets. Gradual progression allows for less blood sugar fluctuation and for changes to be made in medication and meal planning when indicated.

- Consistency is paramount. It is recommended to exercise at the same time of day and at similar intensities, durations, and frequencies. Consistency results in less fluctuation in blood sugar.

- Blood glucose monitoring should be performed more often than normal when first starting an exercise program or when changes are made to the program. Glucose levels can change unpredictably when first beginning physical activity. The regular exerciser will have fewer problems than the occasional, sporadic exerciser. When advising your clients to check their blood glucose levels surrounding exercise, consider the variations in exercise and food intake as well as the risk of postexercise hypoglycemia:

  - Have your client monitor and record his or her blood sugar before, during, and after exercise. In addition, the type, duration, and intensity of exercise should be logged. If food intake varies dramatically, a diet log to track food intake prior to and following exercise should also be kept. A diet log can help to detect extreme swings in blood sugar levels that may be a result of exercise training and allow appropriate diet adjustments to make up for energy expended during the workout. A log of daily blood sugar readings is also a motivational factor when the client notes small, gradual drops in his or her blood sugar.

  - Monitor postexercise blood sugar levels. Hypoglycemia can occur several hours after the end of an exercise session. It is particularly important to check postexercise blood sugar levels when clients increase either the duration or intensity of their exercise programs.

- Avoid isometric exercise or any exercise that results in a sustained increase in systolic BP above 180–200 mmHg. The increase in systolic blood pressure that accompanies high-intensity or isometric exercise is of particular concern to diabetics with microvascular disease. Although there is no direct evidence that high-intensity exercise accelerates the development of diabetic retinopathy or nephropathy, dramatic increases in systolic blood pressure can cause further damage when these diabetic complications are already present. Thus, exercise involving a sustained increase in systolic blood pressure can result in retinal hemorrhage or excess protein in the urine. It is generally advisable that individuals with established microvascular disease of the eye or kidney not engage in any exercise that results in a sustained increase in systolic blood pressure above 180–200 mmHg (Casillas et al. 2007).

All clients with diabetes should keep their physicians informed of their current exercise program, blood sugar readings, and any noted symptoms.

To achieve better health and quality of life, people with diabetes should be encouraged to participate in physical activity regularly. To guide clients with diabetes through an exercise program effectively, the fitness professional must be knowledgeable about the disease. Knowledge of the disease will allow you to:

- Express to your clients the benefits they will receive from exercise.
- Keep your clients safe during and after exercise.
- Understand how your clients' blood glucose levels respond to exercise.
- Create individualized exercise programs that allow your clients to obtain benefits and enjoyment from exercise.

BENEFITS OF EXERCISE

The general benefits of exercise for diabetics are similar to those for nondiabetic populations. In addition, exercise provides some specific benefits for people with diabetes. Exercise has been shown to:

- Lower blood sugar levels and improve the body's ability to use glucose. This is particularly true with T2DM.
- Augment the blood-glucose-lowering effect of injected insulin, thereby reducing the amount of insulin or hypoglycemic medication needed.
- Help reverse the insulin resistance that is associated with excess body fat and is implicated in the etiology of T2DM.
- Delay or prevent the development of atherosclerosis and risk factors related to heart disease, including blood pressure and elevated lipids, which are major threats to people with diabetes.
- Modify body composition and reduce weight when combined with a reduction in caloric intake. Weight loss and exercise increases insulin sensitivity and can allow people with diabetes to reduce the amount of insulin or oral hypoglycemic medication.
- Increase circulation to all parts of the body and therefore lessen the risk for the long-term complication of impaired circulation.
- Play a role in preventing T2DM in people with glucose intolerance, gestational diabetes, or a family history of T2DM.
- Reduce depression, a common occurrence in people with diabetes.
- Reduce stress.

- Allow someone with diabetes to live a "normal life." Some clients may feel limited in exercise by their diabetes, and you can educate them on how to engage in physical activity safely.

RISKS OF EXERCISE

Exercise presents certain risks to clients with diabetes depending on the type and amount of medication they use. The following are areas of risk for clients with diabetes.

Hypoglycemia

Hypoglycemia can occur during or after exercise. Exercise induces glucose utilization, and, therefore, generally a reduction in blood glucose levels, which means that during exercise, your client's blood glucose levels may drop too much. Due to the metabolic effects of exercise, the risk of hypoglycemia does not end with the completion of exercise. Depending on the type and duration of exercise, the risk for late-onset postexercise hypoglycemia can last for up to 30 hours.

Your clients should check his or her blood glucose level prior to an exercise session. If glucose is less than 100 mg/dl, a small amount of carbohydrate should be consumed. Do not start exercise until blood glucose is at least 100 mg/dl. Recent hypoglycemic events will increase the risk of hypoglycemia during exercise (Lisle and Trojian 2006).

Hypoglycemia is a more significant risk for people using insulin than it is for those using oral medications. When exogenous insulin is used, the level of circulating insulin in the body cannot be reduced during exercise even though there is a reduced physiological need for insulin during exercise. The need for insulin is decreased during and after exercise because insulin sensitivity and glucose utilization increases greatly during and after exercise. The injection or infusion site for the insulin is also important. Insulin is absorbed more rapidly when administered to an area close to working muscles. For example, a runner should avoid administering insulin into the thigh before going for a run. Additionally, when insulin levels are high, counter-regulatory hormones that are secreted from the liver to increase blood glucose levels may be impaired. To reduce the risk of hypoglycemia during exercise, encourage your clients to exercise when insulin levels are low (in the morning) or when glucose levels are increasing (following a meal).

It is crucial that you, your client, and the people who surround your client (family, friends, workout buddies) are able to recognize the signs of hypoglycemia and know how to treat it. Unfortunately, your client may not always be able recognize or respond to hypoglycemia; therefore, you and those surrounding your client become important players in keeping your client safe. When hypoglycemia is suspected, your client should check his or her blood glucose levels immediately. Insist that your clients bring their glucose monitor with them to each and every exercise session.

If your client's glucose level is low (<70 mg/dl), stop the exercise and provide him or her with 15 grams of carbohydrate, such as ½ banana, 8 ounces sports drink, or 4 ounces juice (see the list on page 53). Wait for 15 minutes and then have your client check his or her glucose level again. Blood glucose levels should increase about 50 points for 15 grams of carbohydrate. Repeat until glucose levels return to a normal level (70–120 mg/dl) or perhaps higher, depending on the level of insulinization (level of circulating insulin). If the client becomes nonresponsive, or if you are unsure of the actions that need to be taken, call 911. If consciousness drops, oral consumption of glucose may not be an option. A glucose infusion or a glucagon shot may need to be administered by the trainer, an exercise partner, or emergency responder. A glucagon shot increases hepatic glucose production; however, hepatic glycogen stores may be depleted if your client has been engaged in vigorous or long-duration exercise.

In addition to the previous list of symptoms of hypoglycemia, the following are signs of hypoglycemia during exercise:

- Abnormal gait
- Clicking feet when running (kicking feet together, stumbling)
- Lack of balance
- Fatigue, "puniness"
- Confusion
- Seeing stars
- Chills
- Clammy
- Buzzing in ears
- Increased heart rate
- Shaky hands
- Irritability
- Reduction in power (cannot keep up with workout partners or perform at usual level)
- Heart palpitations

Be aware that beta-blocking medication can mask the symptoms of hypoglycemia, such as shakiness and heart palpitations. Clients taking these medications should be closely monitored for hypoglycemic reactions during exercise.

Hyperglycemia

Hyperglycemia can occur during or after exercise. Hyperglycemia is not as an acute risk to your client as hypoglycemia is, unless it progresses to ketoacidosis. Hyperglycemia is most likely to occur after strenuous exercise or in insulin-deficient clients. Insulin deficiency may occur in T2DM or GDM as part of the etiology of the disease when there simply is not enough insulin to bring glucose levels into a normal range due to insulin resistance or impaired insulin function. An insulin-deficient state may also occur in T1DM if the client has not administered enough insulin. Clients with T1DM may put themselves at risk for hyperglycemia from their efforts to reduce the risk of hypoglycemia by either reducing insulin dosages surrounding exercise or by eating too much relative to expenditure or available insulin.

Clients should check their glucose level prior to exercise. If glucose is more than 250 mg/dl, they should check their urine for ketones. If this is not possible, or if glucose is more than 300 mg/dl, they should not initiate exercise.

The signs of hyperglycemia are:

- Dry mouth
- Headache
- Heaviness
- Pressure behind the eyes
- Unusual increase in thirst

Risks Related to Long-Term Complications of Diabetes

People with diabetes are at increased risk of cardiovascular disease and other chronic diseases. Exercise carries inherent cardiovascular risks, such as angina pectoris, myocardial infarction, arrhythmias, sudden death, and increased blood pressure during exercise. Inform your clients of these risks and ensure that they have medical clearance to engage in exercise before initiating an exercise program.

When an individual has additional comorbidities to diabetes, there are additional risks to be aware of when exercising. The following table details the comorbidities and the risks that you will need to be aware of in your clients (Lisle and Trojian 2006).

Comorbidity	Potential Risk with Exercise
Proliferative retinopathy (retinal disease)	Retinal hemorrhage due to increased blood pressure during exercise
Nephropathy (kidney disease)	Fluid imbalances
Peripheral neuropathy (nerve damage in periphery)	Resulting in soft-tissue and joint injuries, predisposition to foot trauma
Autonomic neuropathy (nerve damage in central nervous system)	Results in decreased cardiovascular response to exercise, decreased maximum aerobic capacity, reduced heart rate, impaired response to dehydration, and postural hypotension
Hypertension	Retinal and vitreous hemorrhages

CONTRAINDICATIONS FOR EXERCISE

Hypo- and hyperglycemia and the complications related to diabetes pose risks to exercise participation. In addition, the following are contraindications for exercise for clients with diabetes (Casillas et al. 2007; Pedersen and Saltin 2006):

- Blood glucose >250 mg/dl with ketones
- Blood glucose >300 mg/dl without ketones
- Blood glucose <100 mg/dl
- Unstable angina
- Decompensated heart failure
- Heart rhythm irregularities
- Severe arterial hypertension (blood pressure >180/105 mmHg)
- Recent history of blood clot
- Severe cardio myocardiopathy
- Aortic narrowing
- Orthopedic problems that impair exercise
- Valsalva-like maneuvers and heavy lifting in those with hypertension and active proliferative retinopathy
- Weight-bearing exercise on feet in people with neuropathy and foot ulcers

GLYCEMIA AND EXERCISE: KNOW YOUR CLIENT

Exercise is important in everyone's life. However, it is particularly important if you have diabetes. Exercise can help to control blood sugar levels, maintain desirable weight, increase circulation, and reduce the risk for cardiovascular disease. As a fitness professional working with clients who have diabetes, you understand the benefits and risks associated with exercise. You also need to understand how your client's blood glucose levels will respond to exercise in order to prevent the acute complications of diabetes and exercise.

Keep in mind that individuals with diabetes do not all respond to exercise in the same manner or in the same way as a person without the condition. Several factors affect glucose levels surrounding exercise. Communication with your client is essential for you to be successful in predicting glycemia surrounding exercise. There will be times when glycemia does not follow your predictions, so always be cognizant of the signs of hypo- or hyperglycemia. The most common response is a reduction of blood glucose.

In order to predict a glycemic response and to establish glycemic patterns, you will need to collect information and discuss your client's pre-workout regimen. An understanding of the effects of insulin, food, and exercise on glycemia is crucial to preventing hypo- or hyperglycemia during or after exercise. Individuals with diabetes will see improvements in their performance and experience increased enjoyment in exercise when they are able to avoid the acute complications of their condition surrounding exercise.

Predict a Glycemic Response

The acute response to a single bout of exercise in individuals with diabetes varies. Decreases and increases in blood glucose levels occur. The glycemic response to a single session of exercise is dependent on several factors:

- Blood glucose level prior to exercise
- Intensity, duration, and type of exercise
- Level of circulating insulin (insulinization)
- Food and fluid intake surrounding exercise
- Climate and stress

Of these variables, food and fluid intake, and perhaps insulin dose adjustments, are the easiest to control.

Blood glucose level prior to exercise. The glucose level prior to exercise will affect glycemia during exercise. When blood glucose levels are high, exercise will likely make blood glucose increase further, especially if ketones are present. If glucose levels are low prior to exercise, it will likely continue to drop. For these reasons, it is important to manipulate medications and food intake to achieve as close to normal glycemic levels prior to exercise.

Intensity, duration, and type of exercise. During high-intensity, short-duration exercise (sprints, power sports) there is a risk of hyperglycemia. During this type of exercise, counter-regulatory hormones are released that increase glucose production from the liver. This increase in glucose production may exceed muscle glucose uptake in short-but-intense bouts of exercise.

During low- to moderate-intensity and moderate- to long-duration exercise, hypoglycemia becomes a greater risk. Generally, glucose levels decrease during this type of exercise due to significant muscle glucose uptake. Insulin sensitivity is also greatly increased during and following long-duration exercise. Insulin sensitivity is heightened for at least an hour and up to 30 hours following vigorous or long-duration exercise. Heightened insulin sensitivity means that the need for exogenous insulin is decreased following endurance exercise.

Intermittent, high-intensity exercise (sports) generally lowers glucose levels, but not to the extent seen in continuous, moderate-intensity exercise. In the hours directly following exercise, glucose levels stay relatively stable; however, there is a risk of delayed-onset hypoglycemia because a significant amount of muscle glycogen is used during this type of exercise and will be replenished hours following exercise.

Level of circulating insulin (insulinization). When circulating insulin levels are high, glucose utilization is increased, the use of free fatty acids as an energy source is blocked by insulin, and insulin inhibits the release of counter-regulatory hormones. Therefore, the risk for hypoglycemia is high. If your client is not using exogenous insulin, his or her insulin levels may be normal to high. In the early stages of T2DM and during pre-diabetes, insulin levels tend to be high, although not to the extent that may be seen in T1DM using exogenous insulin. When insulin is administered to the area of working muscles and close to exercise, insulin levels will be higher. Ideally, insulin is administered with adequate time for insulin action to peak prior to initiating exercise. Insulin should be administered away from working muscles.

When circulating insulin levels are low, there is a risk for hyperglycemia surrounding exercise and a risk of ketoacidosis in your T1DM clients. Low levels of insulin may initiate an excessive release of counter-regulatory hormones, which may continue after exercise is completed. When there is inadequate insulin available in T1DM, glucose cannot enter cells, glycemia increases, fat is used as an energy source, and ketones are formed.

Discuss your client's pre-exercise regimen to understand his or her level of insulinization prior to exercise. You need to know the dose and type of insulin administered prior to exercise, the time of insulin administration relative to peak action of insulin, and the time of exercise and the location of insulin administration relative to the type of exercise. Please see chapter 8 for a complete description of insulin type and action.

Food and fluid intake surrounding exercise. During prolonged exercise lasting longer than 60 to 90 minutes, fluid and carbohydrate is needed before, during, and after exercise. If carbohydrates are not appropriately consumed, hypoglycemia becomes a greater risk for all athletes. Carbohydrate is not needed during general exercise lasting less than 60 minutes. Dehydration increases glucose levels as blood volume decreases.

Climate and stress. Warm and hot environments and stress will increase blood glucose levels as well as the risk for illness and infection. As the temperature and/or humidity increases, fluid losses increase. The risk of dehydration becomes greater and your client will have less control over his or her blood glucose. To prevent hyperglycemia, ensure that your clients stay well hydrated and increase insulin dosages if needed. Competition-induced stress can cause an increase in blood glucose levels. The increase can be insignificant or it can lead to hyperglycemia and require a change in medication and/or food intake. If your clients are logging their blood glucose levels surrounding exercise, they will be able to identify this potential increase in blood glucose.

Chronic Response to Exercise

The physiological effects of exercise on glucose metabolism and insulin action results in improvements in glycemic control for those with diabetes. The improvement in glycemic control is believed to be due partly to the accumulative effect of frequent lowering of the blood glucose level with each exercise session. Weight reduction can also contribute to an improvement in glycemic control. Reductions in total daily dose of medications, both oral hypoglycemics and insulin, should be expected. If adjustments are not made in medications, hypoglycemia becomes a greater risk.

As an individual becomes more fit, his or her body will become more efficient and will utilize less glucose during exercise. When glucose utilization during exercise decreases, so does the risk of hypoglycemia. As training duration increases, reductions in insulin dose surrounding exercise need to be adjusted to prevent hyperglycemia.

Establish Glycemic Patterns

In order to improve their performance and enjoyment of exercise encourage your clients with diabetes to use blood glucose, exercise, and food logs. Logs will help them to understand how their body will likely respond to exercise and allow them to make appropriate regimen adjustments. To establish glycemic patterns, your clients should:

- Check and log blood glucose before, during, and after exercise (a continuous glucose monitor is invaluable in providing this information).
- Log food intake and exercise.
- Identify patterns in abnormal values.
- Observe diurnal trends (time of day).

Make Appropriate Regimen Adjustments

Your clients will need to review their food, exercise, and blood glucose logs with their diabetes professional. You can empower them to understand that they can make appropriate regimen changes that will improve their glycemic control surrounding exercise. Only a physician can make changes to medication use and/or dosages. The following are possible regimen changes that may improve glycemic control:

- Level of insulinization surrounding exercise
- Pre-exercise meal
- Pre-exercise insulin adjustments
- During-exercise carbohydrate supplementation
- During-exercise hydration plan
- During-exercise insulin adjustments
- Postexercise carbohydrate supplementation
- Postexercise insulin adjustments

STUDY QUESTIONS

Complete the following questions. The answer key is on pages 119–121.

1. How does exercise effect glucose metabolism?

2. To provide the best exercise program to clients with diabetes what do you need to know?

3. John is apprehensive to start an exercise program. He has type 1 diabetes and is nervous that he may become hypoglycemic when exercising. Describe to John the benefits of starting an exercise program. How would you reassure him that you know what hypoglycemia is, how to recognize it and how to treat it?

4. What are signs of hypoglycemia that are specific to exercise?

5. True or false? All people with diabetes will respond the same to exercise; once you understand how exercise affects glucose levels, you don't need to individualize your recommendations.

6. The glycemic response to a single session of exercise is dependent on several factors, please list these factors.

7. Would you expect blood glucose levels to increase, decrease or stay the same for the following types of exercise:

   a. short duration, high intensity:

   b. low intensity, long duration:

   c. intermittent high intensity (sports):

8. What does insulinization mean?

9. A client with type 2 diabetes is scheduled to see you for personal training on his lunch break. He usually eats at his desk, takes his insulin for his meal and then comes to exercise. Would you expect his insulinization to be relatively high or low?

10. To empower your clients with diabetes, list the regimen changes that may improve glycemic control surrounding exercise.

11. True or false? A medical release is required for any client with diabetes, even if they are in good glycemic control.

12. Do not initiate exercise if blood glucose levels are less than _____ or greater than _____.

13. Case Study: Sally has T1DM and checks her glucose levels 1 hour prior to exercise. Her glucose level is 223 mg/dl. She knows that it is high but is afraid to take insulin before her 30 minute interval workout. What is her likely level of insulinization? What do you expect to happen?

14. Case Study: Tom has T2DM and comes to your 45 minute cardio class. Following class, he comments that the class was particularly hard today. You notice that he has drunk more water than usual and left the class twice for the restroom. What do you suspect and what do you advise him to do?

15. Case Study: It has been a month and John (your apprehensive type 1 client) has established a regular exercise program with you. He attends three personal training sessions each week and does additional cardio two to three times per week. To avoid hypoglycemia, he likely needs to discuss with his physician a _____ in his insulin dose.

5 | EXERCISE DESIGN

Exercise design for a client with diabetes is based on the traditional prescription for developing a training effect in healthy adults. It is, however, modified as indicated by the client's diabetic and general medical status. A thorough medical evaluation and clearance from a physician are necessary before engaging in a physical activity program more intense than walking.

The epidemiologic literature strongly suggests that physical activity prevents T2DM. There is a growing body of support for exercise as a primary strategy in the management of all types of diabetes. Thanks to technology, research, improved medications, and experience, a person with diabetes does not need to be denied the opportunity to participate in and enjoy physical activity. Working with a client who has diabetes can provide many challenges, as well as rewards, for both the fitness practitioner and the client.

EXERCISE PROGRAM DEVELOPMENT

The American Diabetes Association and American Heart Association support the Physical Activity Guidelines for Americans (United States Department of Health and Human Services 2009) for individuals with diabetes who do not have medical contraindications (ACSM 2010; Buse et al. 2007; Sigal et al. 2006). In addition, in 2010 the American College of Sports Medicine (ACSM) and the American Diabetes Association issued exercise guidelines for T2DM as a Joint Position Statement, which was published in the journals *Medicine and Science in Sports and Exercise* and *Diabetes Care.* The new guidelines call for both aerobic and resistance training exercise and provide specific advice for people with diabetes who might be limited from engaging in vigorous exercise.

The position statement states that:

- Exercise plays a major role in the prevention and control of insulin resistance, prediabetes, gestational diabetes mellitus (GDM), T2DM, and diabetes-related health complications and can assist with cardiovascular risk, mortality, and quality of life.
- Physical activity is critical for optimal health in individuals with T2DM.
- Exercise must be undertaken regularly to have continued benefits.

- Both aerobic exercise and resistance training should be included in exercise programming for diabetes management.

To view the complete *Exercise and Type 2 Diabetes: American College of Sports Medicine and the American Diabetes Association: Joint Position Statement* visit:
http://journals.lww.com/acsm-msse/Fulltext/2010/12000/Exercise_and_Type_2_Diabetes__American_College_of.18.aspx

The 2009 Physical Activity Guidelines for Americans as published by the U.S. Department of Health and Human Services are:

Frequency:
- At least 3 days per week and as much as every day of the week.
- Avoid more than 2 consecutive days of physical inactivity per week.

Duration and intensity:
- At least 150 minutes per week of moderate-intensity aerobic physical activity (40–60% of maximal oxygen consumption [VO_2max] or 50–70% of maximum heart rate) and/or at least 90 minutes per week of vigorous aerobic exercise (above 60% VO_2max or above 70% maximum heart rate).
- Moderate-to-vigorous aerobic and/or resistance exercise should be performed 5 or more hours per week as it is associated with greater cardiovascular disease risk reduction compared with lower volumes of physical activity.
- For long-term maintenance of major weight loss (30 lb or more), more exercise (7 hours per week of moderate or vigorous aerobic activity) may be helpful.

Resistance training:
- In the absence of contraindications, perform resistance exercise 2–3 times per week, targeting all major muscle groups and progress to 3 sets of 8–10 repetitions at a weight that cannot be lifted more than 8–10 times. Initial supervision and periodic reassessment by a qualified exercise specialist is recommended.

Older adult:
- If at risk for falling, perform exercise that maintains or improves balance.
- Older adults (aged 65 years and older) are encouraged to follow these guidelines or be as active as physical limitations allow.

The 2010 ACSM/ADA guidelines for both aerobic and resistance training include the following:

Aerobic exercise guidelines:
Frequency:
- At least 3 times a week; preferably up to 5 times a week.

- No more than 2 consecutive days between bouts (due to transient nature of exercise on insulin action).

Intensity:
- 40–60% of VO_2max (moderate intensity); greater health benefits can be achieved at >60% of VO_2max.
- Physical activity above the recommended amount of intensity provides even greater health benefits.
- Exercise intensity predicts improvements in blood glucose control greater than increases in exercise volume.
- Increase exercise intensity as tolerated.

Duration:
- 150 minutes or more per week; performed in bouts of 10 minutes or more.

Mode:
- Exercise that uses the large muscle groups of the body.

Progression:
- More gradually for some individuals with T2DM and clients with cardiovascular, orthopedic, and other physical limitations.

Resistance training guidelines:

Frequency:
- At least 2 times per week on nonconsecutive days.
- Progress to 3 times a week.

Intensity:
- Initially at 50% of 1 Repetition Maximum (1RM): 10–15 RM.
- Gradually increase to 75–80% of 1RM; 8–10 RM.
- Strength exercise machines or free weights can be used; both have shown equivalent benefits for blood glucose control.

Mode:
- 5–10 resistance training exercises of the major muscle groups. The majority of studies with resistance training and diabetic subjects train the gluteals, thighs, chest, back, core, shoulders, and arms.

Progression:
- For greater blood glucose control, gradually increase with heavier weights first versus doing more sets.
- Start with 1 set per exercise and progress to 2–3 sets.
- If training 2 times per week, progress gradually to 3 times per week.
- The optimal goal for the client is to achieve:
  - 3 times per week of resistance training.
  - 3 sets of 8–10 repetitions at 75–80% of 1RM per exercise (train to momentary muscular fatigue).
  - Train the major muscle groups of the body.

Due to potentially complex physical limitations of the diabetic client, the ACSM and ADA recommend that clients with diabetes always be properly supervised by a qualified exercise trainer when engaged in resistance training. This will help to ensure optimal blood glucose management and other health benefits while minimizing the risk of injury.

Exercise for the client with diabetes should always be individually designed and appropriate with respect to mode, intensity, duration, frequency, and progression of exercise. In general, consistency in all exercise parameters is crucial to maintain blood glucose homeostasis. No two individuals with diabetes will respond to exercise in exactly the same way. Individual adjustment based on physical status, ability, and exercise tolerance will be required for each client. The combined benefits of resistance training and aerobic exercise in diabetic populations versus aerobic only or resistance only training include better improvement in A1c, better management and prevention of T2DM, and increased weight loss.

Mode

Aerobic exercise, strength training, and flexibility exercise are indicated for individuals with diabetes. Continuous large-muscle exercise such as walking, bicycling, swimming, rowing, stair climbing, and group dance is appropriate. Aerobic exercise reduces the risk of cardiovascular disease, enhances glycemic control, and assists in achieving or maintaining a healthy body weight. Upper-extremity exercise performed with the arm ergometer can be used for clients who cannot tolerate lower-extremity activity. Non-weight-bearing activities are better suited to clients with peripheral neuropathy. Cross-training may help to reduce musculoskeletal problems and the pain brought on by neuropathy to the lower extremities and may help to increase comfort and exercise compliance.

Individuals who are sedentary may initially engage in entry-level exercise by participating in enjoyable lifestyle activities such as gardening, yard work, housework, dancing, walking, and taking the stairs. As they gain strength and endurance by participating in these activities, their ability to enjoy planned aerobic exercise will increase. Pleasurable activities increase compliance. Encourage clients starting a new program to exercise with friends or family members. This also helps to ensure safety during exercise.

Intensity

The selection of exercise intensity for people with diabetes is similar to that for healthy adults. In general, moderate-intensity exercise is recommended. Lower-intensity exercise may increase the acceptability of exercise by deconditioned or elderly clients with low exercise capabilities.

Exercise intensity is one factor associated with a hypoglycemic response and may determine the magnitude of the fall in blood glucose with exercise in individuals with diabetes. High-intensity exercise appears to accentuate the glucose-lowering effect on insulin to a greater degree than low-intensity exercise of the same duration; however, the risk of hypoglycemia is also increased with prolonged exercise duration (American Diabetes Association 2002). The 2010 ACSM/ADA position paper states that "physical activity above the recommended amount of intensity provides even great health benefits." It is important to note that exercise intensity predicts improvements in blood glucose control greater than increases in exercise volume.

Consistency of workload and frequency of exercise are important variables for your clients when designing exercise. Regular and moderately paced exercise may be a better choice for clients with diabetes than exercise that varies in intensity.

Clients who have been unable to be physically active due to illness, poor health, or medical conditions and are returning to exercise may require several days to several weeks to regain their original exercise workloads. They should begin activity at a lesser intensity and gradually progress to higher exercise levels. This is particularly the case with the client who has cardiovascular, othorpedic, or metabolic disease. Re-entry at too rapid a pace can easily trigger a relapse.

Exercising at higher intensities may be appropriate for clients with capabilities to achieve higher fitness levels and are motivated by higher fitness goals or vocational requirements. The exercise prescription for intensity, mode, frequency, and duration should be based on your clinical judgment of safety and your client's goals and needs.

Duration

The entry-level client may need to begin with exercise durations of 5 to 10 minutes and progress to 30 to 60 minutes of continuous or intermittent exercise to accumulate the minimum recommended duration of 150 minutes a week of physical activity. Intermittent exercise works particularly well with extremely deconditioned individuals, as well as with those with peripheral vascular disease, intermittent claudication, or neuropathy in the lower extremities. Intermittent exercise may help clients avoid excessive oxygen debt or fatigue and may also permit a greater total workload at each exercise session before the occurrence of activity-limiting symptoms, such as leg pain.

The duration of the activity is correlated with the magnitude of the decrease in blood sugar levels in both type 1 and type 2 diabetes. This means that 40 minutes of stationary cycling at 50% to 55% of VO_2max produces a significantly greater blood glucose lowering effect than 20 minutes of cycling at the same intensity.

Frequency

Aim for consistency in the frequency of exercise, as well as consistency of duration and intensity. A moderate-intensity workout performed five to seven days per week is optimal for consistency. It also maximizes caloric expenditure of 2,000 kcal or more a week required for weight management. However, most beginning exercisers will begin with two to three days of exercise per week and progress to the desired frequency.

To assist in achieving consistency in frequency, it is recommended to exercise at approximately the same time of day. Remember, consistency means fewer fluctuations in blood glucose levels.

Progression

Exercise should be progressed slowly and as tolerated by the client. Only one exercise variable should be changed at a time. Exercise that is progressed gradually allows for less blood glucose fluctuation. Many clients with T2DM have cardiovascular, orthopedic, and other physical limitations. Exercise design must progress more gradually for these individuals. Strenuous exercise can worsen diabetes-related problems such as eye, kidney, and nerve damage. For example, eye problems can be worsened by performing exercises that involve straining, such as weightlifting. In addition, excessive walking or running can aggravate pain from nerve damage or poor circulation to the feet.

In general, once your client has obtained a continuous and sustainable duration of exercise and if your client is tolerating the exercise intensity, gradually increase the intensity of exercise first and then the duration and frequency of exercise. Remember that exercise intensity predicts improvement in blood glucose greater than increases in total volume.

Heart rate, perceived exertion, physical observation by the practitioner, and client indication can all be used to determine when it is appropriate to increase workload. A person with diabetes who progresses too quickly can worsen diabetes-related problems and decrease enjoyment in exercise.

To avoid injury when progressing resistance training exercises, increases in weight or resistance are undertaken first and only when the target number of repetitions per set can be exceeded consistently, followed by a greater number of sets, and lastly by increased training frequency.

Assigning Initial Workloads

Assigning initial workloads for aerobic exercise is not an exact science. Continual and progressive refinement is necessary to find the workload that best suits each client. Fitness evaluations or graded exercise test (GXT) results can be used to assist in determining initial workloads. Clients with cardiovascular disease or who are at risk for cardiovascular disease may benefit from a cardiac stress test prior to engaging in physical activity. Consult with your client's physician if you have any concerns regarding the safety of exercise participation or progression. A typical approach for assigning beginning workloads is to start the client with exercise that he or she can sustain with reasonable comfort for 10 minutes. The duration or intensity of exercise can be increased from there according to client tolerance.

Resistance Training

Aerobic activity alone cannot provide the full benefits of exercise to the individual with diabetes. Recent research has shown that strength training is as important as—and perhaps more important than—aerobic training in managing diabetes. The most recent studies have reinforced the additional benefit of combining aerobic and resistance training for people with diabetes. Resistance, or strength, training exercise should be encouraged in all of your clients with diabetes. Much of the effect of physical activity appears to be due to the metabolic adaptation of skeletal muscle (Buse et al. 2007; Sigal et al. 2006). Resistance training improves muscular strength and endurance and functional ability, which is important for all ages, particularly older adults. Strength training also improves bone health and balance, thereby reducing the risk of falls and bone fractures.

Studies related to strength training with exercise machines and free weights have shown equivalent benefits for blood glucose control. Rubberized resistance tubes and bands, wrist and ankle cuff weights, wall pulleys, weighted bars or balls, and dumbbells also can be used. Work with your client to ensure that your recommendations match their expectations of accessibility to equipment.

In general, resistance training is safe and effective for most people with diabetes provided you follow the recommended guidelines. However, heavy weightlifting should be avoided for clients who have severe neuropathy and diabetes-related eye problems. People with proliferative diabetic retinopathy should not participate in resistance training. The following guidelines are recommended when working with clients who have diabetes (American Heart Association 2007; ACSM/ADA 2010):

- Begin with 1 set of 10–15 repetitions for all major muscles groups. Fewer repetitions may be appropriate. The weight load is based on the client's goals, medical status, and tolerance. Sets can be increased gradually from 1 to 3. Repetitions may decrease to 6–8 or 8–10 repetitions per set as weight load increases. Total workout time is a consideration.
- Progress the client as indicated by 5% when 12–15 reps can be accomplished comfortably.
- Increase weight only when the target number of repetitions per set can be exceeded consistently. This is followed by an increase in number of sets and lastly by increased training frequency.
- For greater blood glucose control, gradually progress with heavier weights first versus doing more set.
- Avoid straining and breath holding. Exhale during the exertion phase of the lift.
- Raise the weights in slow, controlled movements and emphasize full range of motion when lifting.
- Exercise large muscle groups before small muscle groups and include lower, upper, and core body exercises.

- Strength train 2–3 times per week.
- Loosely hold handgrips when possible. Sustained tight gripping may evoke an excessive blood pressure response.
- Avoid placing resistance bands or tubing around the legs and feet, especially in clients with diabetic neuropathy.
- Stop the exercise if warning signs or symptoms of hypoglycemia, dizziness, arrhythmia, unusual shortness of breath, or angina are present.

The ACSM and ADA recommend that clients with diabetes always be properly supervised by a qualified exercise trainer when engaged in resistance training. This will help to ensure optimal blood glucose management and other health benefits while minimizing the risk of injury.

It may take six months to a year for your client to attain the aerobic and resistance training goals. It has been show that A1c improvements are better with the combined exercise program of aerobic exercise and resistance training. Combining a healthy eating plan with the aerobic and resistance training exercise will result in optimal weight loss, improved blood glucose management, and better health for the client with diabetes.

STUDY QUESTIONS

Complete the following questions. The answer key is on page 121.

1. How much aerobic and resistance training exercise is recommended by the American College of Sports Medicine and the American Diabetes Associations per week?

2. What long-term complication would prevent someone from engaging in a regular strength training program?

3. Case Study: Briefly describe differences in the mode, duration, frequency, intensity of exercise that you could recommend for these two clients.

   a. Leonora, 78 years old, type 2 diabetes for 28 years, is new to exercise and has peripheral neuropathy. Her goal is to improve energy level and overall quality of life by engaging in exercise.

   b. Jim, 38 years old, type 1 diabetes for 10 years, no complications, currently exercises three times a week for twenty minutes and wants to improve fitness.

6 | NUTRITION SURROUNDING EXERCISE

An awareness of food and fluid intake before, during, and after exercise and the glycemic response to exercise is crucial for the safety of your clients with diabetes. Adjustments in carbohydrate intake surrounding exercise have the most profound effects on maintaining glycemic control.

Carbohydrate increases blood glucose levels. Too much carbohydrate consumed before, during, or after exercise can result in hyperglycemia. Too little increases the risk of hypoglycemia. The amount of carbohydrate needed depends on the mode, intensity, and duration of exercise. Carbohydrate needs increase during higher-intensity and longer-duration exercise.

Clients will be interested in what to eat and drink before, during, and after exercise. Provide your clients with the following guidance, along with a referral to a registered dietitian who specializes in diabetes and/or sports nutrition.

BEFORE EXERCISE

All individuals with diabetes should be encouraged to consume at least a small amount of carbohydrate prior to exercise to avoid exercising on an empty stomach. Ideally, the client should eat a meal or snack 1 to 3 hours before exercising. The size of this meal should increase as the duration or intensity of exercise increases. For example, ½ cup cereal with 1 cup milk and fruit would be satisfactory for a 30- to 45-minute bout of exercise. A piece of toast with marmalade can be added for a 60- to 90-minute workout. A carbohydrate-rich snack containing 15 to 30 grams of carbohydrate, such as a banana, 8- to 16-ounce sports drink, or 1 cup yogurt, can be consumed 15 to 30 minutes before starting endurance exercise or if blood glucose levels are less than 100 mg/dl.

Your clients should be well hydrated prior to the start of exercise. The best way to assess hydration is to notice urine color and odor. Urine that has a dark color and/or strong odor indicates dehydration. To prevent starting exercise in a dehydrated state, the American College of Sports Medicine (2010) recommends that approximately 16 to 24 ounces of fluids be consumed slowly in the hours prior to initiating exercise. To avoid dehydration during endurance exercise lasting longer than 60 to 90 minutes, 16 ounces of fluids 1 to 2 hours prior to exercise, plus 8 ounces immediately before exercise is recommended.

DURING EXERCISE

Water is sufficient during continuous exercise that is less than 60 to 90 minutes in duration. When the duration of exercise increases, carbohydrate and electrolytes are required during exercise. Suggest that your clients carry some form of quick-acting sugar during exercise in case of a hypoglycemic reaction and extra carbohydrate during longer-endurance bouts of exercise. Lifesavers, hard candy, glucose tablets, fruit juice, and sports products work well. Blood glucose levels should be monitored during exercise. Adjustments in the amount of carbohydrate may be made during exercise to prevent hyper- or hypoglycemia.

Recommend to your clients that they ingest 15 to 30 grams of CHO every 15 to 30 minutes for a total of 30 to 75 grams per hour during moderate-intensity exercise lasting longer than 60 to 90 minutes (ADA and ACSM 2000). Fluid, from water or sports drinks, should be consumed at a rate of 4 to 10 ounces every 15 minutes for a total of at least 24 ounces per hour (ADA and ACSM 2000). Ideally, your client will customize his or her fluid intake based on sweat rate (ACSM 2007). Typically, sports products are used to provide fluid, carbohydrate, and electrolytes. Foods such as bananas, granola bars, and figs can also be used in conjunction with water to provide carbohydrate, electrolytes, and fluids.

AFTER EXERCISE

Encourage all individuals to consume at least a small snack and water following exercise to promote rehydration and muscle recovery. Increased consumption of fluids, electrolytes, carbohydrate, and protein are required following endurance exercise. A balanced meal or snack containing carbohydrate and protein should be consumed immediately following endurance exercise. Food should be consumed every 2 hours following prolonged endurance exercise lasting longer than 2 to 3 hours. At least 16 to 24 ounces of fluids should be consumed following exercise, or 16 to 24 ounces per pound of body weight lost during exercise (ACSM 2007).

Monitor postexercise blood glucose to determine if dietary intake is appropriate. Be alert for postexercise hypoglycemia. Clients who use insulin have the greatest risk of developing severe hypoglycemia 6 to 14 hours after strenuous exercise when blood glucose levels can continue to decrease. It can take the body up to 24 hours to replace the glycogen that was used during the workout. Muscle and hepatic (liver) glycogen must be restored postexercise during periods of rest. Avoid alcohol around the time of exercise as it can promote hypoglycemia.

TREATING HYPOGYLCEMIA

If your client experiences hypoglycemia during exercise, you must know how to respond appropriately. If you or your client notice any signs of hypoglycemia, check blood glucose levels. If glucose is less than 70 mg/dl, stop exercise and provide a carbohydrate-rich food. Follow the 15–50 rule: 15 grams of carbohydrate will increase blood glucose approximately 50 points in 15 minutes.

Examples of 15 grams carbohydrate

- 4 oz fruit juice
- 8 oz sports drink
- 8 oz regular soda
- ½ banana
- 1 Fig Newton
- ¾ sports gel (such as Gu)
- 2 sports chews (such as Cliff Shot Bloks)
- 3 Life Savers candies

HYDRATION

Dehydration is a concern when working with clients with diabetes. People with diabetes have a greater risk of dehydration due to the increased fluid requirement of the kidneys and urine output needed to flush excess glucose from the body if their glucose levels tend to remain above normal. Follow these steps to prevent dehydration in the physically active client with diabetes (ADA and ACSM 2000):

- Drink plenty of fluids each day.
- Drink cool uncarbonated water before, during, and after exercise:
    - 20 oz or 2½ cups (600 ml) 2 hours before exercise
    - 8–16 oz (250–500 ml) 30 minutes before exercise
    - 4 oz (90–160 ml) every 15 minutes during exercise
    - As indicated by body weight and symptoms after exercise
    - Drink to satisfy thirst; don't force yourself to drink more
- Recognize the symptoms of dehydration:
    - Severe thirst
    - Dizziness
    - Tachycardia
    - Confusion
    - Headache
    - Irritability

- Weigh self before and after exercise:
  - A loss of more than 2% body weight indicates dehydration
  - To rehydrate, consume 16–24 ounces per pound of body weight lost
- Monitor urine volume and color: A small amount of dark urine may be a sign of dehydration

STUDY QUESTIONS

Complete the following questions. The answer key is on pages 121–122.

1. Describe the 15–50 rule.

2. Case Study: Rebecca is going for a 3 mile run (she runs about 10–11-minute miles) on Saturday morning. What do recommend she eat and drink before, during and after exercise?

3. Case Study: What do you recommend Rebecca eat and drink before, during, and after a 90-minute bike ride?

7 | SPECIAL CONSIDERATIONS FOR DIABETES AND EXERCISE

Specific considerations for the various types of diabetes are necessary to keep your clients safe and to progress them in their exercise program. Each type of diabetes comes with different variables for you to consider. Athletes and older adults also have unique needs.

CLIENTS USING INSULIN

Clients who use insulin offer a greater challenge for prescribing appropriate exercise because their treatment requires exogenous insulin. With most types of exercise these individuals must adjust insulin dosage or carbohydrate intake before, during, and after exercise to maintain normal glycemic control and to avoid hypoglycemia. People who use insulin should not exercise alone, and personal trainers, fitness instructors, exercise partners, and teammates should be aware of the individual's condition and be able to respond to an insulin reaction. Encourage your clients who use insulin always to carry a diabetic identification when exercising.

Exercise may affect your clients using insulin differently from those who do not use insulin; therefore, it is important to consider these guidelines when planning a program for these clients.

Glycemic Control

Blood glucose levels must be under good control prior to exercise. If blood glucose levels are not well controlled, it is difficult to predict the body's response to exercise. When insulin deficiency is severe and diabetes control poor, hepatic glucose production and the breakdown of fat to ketones may exceed the ability of the muscles to use them. As a result, blood glucose levels increase and ketones accumulate. Conversely, when there is an excess of insulin, the hormones responsible for stimulating hepatic glucose production are inhibited and hypoglycemia becomes a risk.

The most common risk of exercise for people with T1DM is hypoglycemia. Consumption of carbohydrate-rich foods is advised prior to exercise and after exercise for your clients using insulin in order to prevent hypoglycemia. Insulin that is taken with these foods

57

should be adjusted appropriately. The amount of carbohydrate that should be consumed will vary depending on glucose level, insulinization, and exercise intensity and duration. Skipping meals to avoid insulin is not effective and will lead to poor performance. During endurance exercise, carbohydrate must be consumed to prevent hypoglycemia. Postexercise and nighttime hypoglycemia can be prevented by exercising earlier in the day and by reducing insulin dosages after completing exercise. Encourage your clients to check their blood glucose level at bedtime and during the night if exercise intensity or volume is high.

Monitoring Blood Glucose

Monitor blood glucose closely. Close monitoring of all associated factors is imperative for people using insulin. These clients should monitor and log blood glucose levels, insulin dosage, amount and type of food eaten, and exercise performed. During endurance exercise, monitor blood glucose every 30 minutes. Monitoring provides specific information that will indicate the nutritional and medication adjustments needed to maintain blood glucose control.

The following are contraindications based on blood glucose levels (ADA 2002). In general, the client should not exercise if the blood glucose level is less than 100 mg/dl prior to exercise. If the blood glucose level is above 250 mg/dl prior to exercise, the client should check his or her urine for ketones. Do not allow the client to exercise if ketones are present or if blood glucose is above 300 mg/dl. Exercise may increase the risk of ketoacidosis and coma.

Insulin Adjustments

Exercise increases glucose utilization and insulin sensitivity; therefore, reductions in insulin dosage should be considered. Often, insulin dosages need to be reduced on the day of exercise. While it is outside your scope of practice to recommend changes in medications or make specific recommendations for target glucose levels, you are in an important position to help your client establish optimal glycemic control. Reductions in insulin dose may occur before, during, or after exercise. The amount of the reduction varies depending on the individual's insulin sensitivity, the duration and intensity of the exercise, the time of day, glucose level prior to exercise, and foods consumed. Self-testing of blood glucose is critical and should be the basis for every adjustment with insulin dosage. Engaging in exercise at the same time of day, with similar intensity and duration, will assist in regulating insulin dosages. Possible insulin adjustments that your client could discuss with his or her physician or diabetes educator are (Colberg 2009):

- Rapid/fast-acting bolus before exercise: reduce by 10–30% and up to 70–90% before endurance exercise.
- Rapid/fast-acting bolus after exercise: reduce by 20–50%.

- Long-acting insulin or pump basal rate before, during, and after exercise: reduce by 10–50%.

All insulin adjustments should be discussed with the healthcare provider.

Insulin injection sites prior to and during exercise will affect insulinization during exercise. Use sites that will not be exercised vigorously during the workout. Exercise accelerates the mobilization of insulin from subcutaneous deposits, which can result in hyperinsulinemia and can inhibit hepatic glucose production. For example, walking and jogging greatly increase the absorption of insulin from the legs. Insulin will be absorbed more slowly if it is injected into the stomach or arm. The abdomen is a good site for insulin injections prior to lower-body exercise. If intense abdominal work is to be performed, an alternative site should be used.

Avoid exercise at the time of peak insulin effect. Time of peak insulin action depends on the type of insulin: long, intermediate, short, or rapid acting. See the section in chapter 8 that details types of insulin. Time exercise to miss peak periods of administered insulin. In general, insulin should be injected more than 1 hour before the start of physical activity to avoid a hypoglycemic effect. Ideally, insulin levels will be low during exercise, for example in the morning or 2 to 3 hours following a dose of fast- or rapid-acting insulin.

CLIENTS USING ORAL MEDICATIONS AND/OR LIFESTYLE MODIFICATION

This population of clients will likely be prediabetic or have GDM or T2DM. They may be new to exercise, overweight, deconditioned, or resistant to exercise. Their motivation for exercise likely will be to prevent diabetes or to prevent complications from diabetes. The exercise prescription for these clients will be similar to those who do not have diabetes. Educate your clients on the benefits of exercise and its role in promoting glycemic control, insulin sensitivity, and weight management.

Glycemic Control

These clients are not at risk for ketoacidosis; however, exercising with elevated blood glucose levels greater than 250 mg/dl is still detrimental. Encourage your clients to check their glucose level prior to exercise. When glucose levels are above normal (>120 mg/dl), the risk for dehydration and early fatigue increases. Exercise and hydration are effective ways to bring glucose into a normal range.

Insulin levels are generally lower in this population and, therefore, these individuals may experience hyperglycemia more frequently than hypoglycemia as a result of exercise. During exercise, counter-regulatory hormones and glucagon are released and stimulate hepatic glucose output. Hepatic glucose production may be excessive, resulting in hyperglycemia following exercise. Fear of and frustration from hyperglycemia may discourage individuals from engaging in exercise. Encourage continued participation in exercise and consider lower-intensity exercise that will result in less hepatic stimulation.

Oral Medications

The impact of oral hypoglycemic agents on exercise is minimal, with the exception of medications that stimulate the pancreas to secrete more insulin. See the section in chapter 8 that details the classes of oral medications.

CLIENTS WITH GESTATIONAL DIABETES

Current research indicates that exercise can reduce the risk of GDM progressing to T2DM by improving blood glucose during pregnancy, normalizing weight gain during pregnancy, and promoting weight loss following pregnancy (Ceysens, Rouiller, and Boulvain 2006). Exercise should be encouraged during pregnancy, even if the woman has GDM. Special medical clearance should be obtained prior to starting an exercise program.

Contraindications for Exercise with GDM and Warning Signs to Terminate Exercise

Absolute contraindications (ACSM 2010):

- Significant heart disease
- Restrictive lung disease
- Incompetent cervix or cervical cerclage
- Pregnant with multiples
- Risk of preterm labor
- Premature labor
- Persistent bleeding during second or third trimester
- Placenta previa
- Ruptured membranes
- Pregnancy-induced hypertension

Relative contraindications (ACSM 2010):

- Maternal cardiac arrhythmia
- Fetal intrauterine growth restriction
- History of sedentary lifestyle
- Orthopedic limitations
- Uncontrolled hypertension
- Uncontrolled diabetes
- Uncontrolled seizure disorder
- Uncontrolled hyperthyroidism

- Chronic bronchitis
- Smoking

Warning signs to terminate exercise during pregnancy (ACSM 2010):
- Vaginal bleeding
- Leakage of amniotic fluid
- Preterm labor
- Decreased fetal movement
- Chest pain, shortness of breath/labored breathing before exertion
- Headache, dizziness, muscle weakness
- Calf pain or swelling

ATHLETES WITH DIABETES

Athletes who participate in sports and vigorous training need to be able to juggle insulin, food, and their training continually to challenge the limits of their athletic abilities safely. Fortunately, blood glucose monitoring makes it possible to make routine adjustments to maintain the delicate blood glucose balance of food, insulin, and activity. However, every individual is different, and any strenuous athletic endeavor or change in the diabetic management plan should be discussed with the individual's healthcare team.

Nutrition for the Athlete with Diabetes

Nutritional guidelines for the athlete with diabetes are similar to athletes who do not have diabetes: carbohydrate and fluids must be consumed before, during, and after exercise. Blood glucose monitoring before, during, and after long training or events will assist the individual in identifying how much additional carbohydrates to ingest and what insulin adjustments to make in different situations. An exercise log is a good tool to help the athlete with diabetes make decisions about food, insulin, and activity. Instruct the athlete to record insulin injection times and amount, blood glucose results, and comments about the exercise intensity and duration, how the exercise felt, and any other pertinent changes. The athlete also should keep track of insulin reactions and how much food was needed to treat them.

Before Exercise

The athlete should eat at a balanced carbohydrate meal 1 to 3 hours before exercise, such as whole-grain toast, fruit, and eggs or cereal, fruit, and milk. Another small carbohydrate-rich snack may be needed immediately before a long-endurance activity, such as a banana, cup of yogurt, or energy bar. Check glucose level and adjust food and insulin appropriately. Ensure that your client is adequately hydrated.

Athletes who wear an insulin pump may take the pump off prior to contact sports or swimming. Their glucose level will initially drop due to increased glucose utilization during exercise; however, their glucose level may begin to increase after 1 hour without the administration of exogenous insulin. Therefore, exogenous insulin should be given hourly during exercise (Lisle and Trojian 2006). Frequent blood glucose monitoring is required when the insulin pump is removed to avoid hyperglycemia.

During Exercise

Encourage your athlete to consume 30 to 75 grams of carbohydrate per hour depending on glucose level, body size, exercise intensity, and exercise duration. Encourage the intake of 100 to 500 milligrams sodium and at least 24 ounces fluids per hour of endurance exercise. For exercise lasting less than 60 to 90 minutes, plain water is sufficient.

Because glucose can enter the cells more readily during vigorous exercise, blood sugar may drop quickly. Hypoglycemic responses during intense training should be monitored closely. When glucose stores are low, the brain feels the insult, and motor coordination can be affected. Signs of severe hypoglycemia are disorientation, acting drunk, and stumbling. When hypoglycemia is suspected, check blood glucose levels and treat blood glucose levels less than 70 mg/dl with fruit juices, oral glucose tablets, or sports drinks/products. Use these readily available carbohydrate sources to quickly increase glucose levels. Once glucose returns to normal, a small snack containing carbohydrate, fat, and protein (such as an energy bar or peanut butter sandwich) will prevent glucose levels from falling. If glucose levels are less than 50 mg/dl, treat glucose level and terminate exercise. Monitoring glucose, adjusting insulin, and consuming carbohydrate before, during, and after a long exercise session are important strategies to prevent hypoglycemia.

Another concern during exercise is insulin pumps, which can malfunction or become dislodged during exercise. Without insulin infusion the risk of ketoacidosis is high. Jostling and movement during exercise can negatively affect the infusion site or kink the catheter. Sweating can also dislodge the infusion site. Additionally, insulin is heat sensitive: the pump contains insulin and body heat needs to be considered during exercise to maintain the effectiveness of the insulin (Lisle and Trojian 2006).

After Exercise

In the 15 to 30 minutes following vigorous or endurance exercise the body actively replenishes muscle glycogen, and carbohydrate needs are high. Hypoglycemia is a risk following exercise due to glycogen replacement. A carbohydrate-rich snack that contains some protein, such as fruit and yogurt smoothie, cereal and milk, chocolate milk, or a turkey sandwich, should be consumed immediately following exercise. Protein enhances muscle recovery and promotes glycogen storage. Fluids should be encouraged, as this is also the optimal time for rehydration. Another carbohydrate-rich meal should be consumed 2 hours after endurance exercise.

Clients should continue to test blood glucose every 2 hours for the next 12 hours to determine fluctuations in glycemia and to prevent hypoglycemia. Repeat this procedure several times to understand how the body is responding to the exercise. If blood glucose is below normal ranges, increase caloric intake for 12 to 24 hours after exercise. This procedure should be repeated any time a major change in the intensity or duration of the training occurs. Early warning signs of hypoglycemia following exercise include exhaustion, weakness, and increase in appetite. Increased calorie intake, particularly from carbohydrates, and reductions in insulin help to prevent postexercise hypoglycemia. Frequent glucose checks will avoid hyper- and hypoglycemia. Athletes often must use a trial-and-error method to fine-tune diet, medication, and exercise when participating in intense training regimes and competition.

Insulin Adjustments

Many insulin adjustments are available to your client to improve glycemic control, enjoyment of exercise, and athletic performance. Reductions in insulin before, during, and after exercise should be considered. Ensure that your clients are aware of these potential adjustments and encourage them to discuss regimen changes with their healthcare provider. Remember that adjustments made for one individual may not work for another. Athletes must be aware constantly of the signals that indicate insulin reaction and have an appropriate treatment plan.

Tool Kit for Athletes with Diabetes

The following is a list of supplies that your athletes with diabetes, especially those using insulin, need to keep available during exercise. For athletes who travel, plans need to be made in advance to ensure that these supplies are available. Extra supplies are necessary when traveling.

- Insulin and/or oral medications (plus extra)
- Blood glucose monitor
- Blood glucose test strips
- Batteries
- Lancets
- Insulin pump supplies (plus 1–2 extras) or needles
- Carbohydrate source: sports gel, glucose tabs, or carton(s) of juice
- Glucagon shot
- Ice pack to keep insulin cool (if needed)
- Alcohol swabs

Individuals with diabetes can participate in all types of sports. High-risk sports such as parachuting, hang-gliding, or scuba diving previously were not recommended for T1DM athletes. However, with skilled training, individuals with diabetes may be able to participate in these activities. Make sure coaches, teammates, and colleagues know of the athlete's condition and how to treat an insulin reaction. By learning how the body responds to the physical stress of training and competition, each athlete can reach his or her full potential.

OLDER CLIENTS WITH DIABETES

Exercise participation for older adults (65 years and older) improves quality of life and health. Regular participation in physical activity has been shown to lower healthcare costs, lower hospitalization rate, and prevent and/or slow the progression of chronic disease (Nguyen et al. 2008). Aging is associated with the development of impaired glucose tolerance. It is unknown exactly how much of this impaired glucose tolerance is a primary effect of aging and how much is secondary to other frequently associated age-related changes such as increased adipose tissue, decreased muscle mass, and decreased physical activity. Diet and exercise play a significant role in preventing the age-associated decline in glucose tolerance and have been shown to effectively delay the development of diabetes by 71% in people aged 60 and over (NIDDK 2001). Exercise is important for all older adults to improve quality of life and maintain an independent lifestyle. Increased physical activity has been demonstrated to provide a protective benefit to prevent the development of T2DM in older adults (Tuomilheto et al. 2001).

In a nationwide survey of 9,156 SilverSneakers members, 14% reported having diabetes. Forty-one percent of the diabetic members reported improved health after one or more years of participation in the SilverSneakers program, and 46% reported improved body weight. High-risk sedentary behavior was reduced by 59% (Healthways 2007).

Special considerations are necessary when working with older adults who have diabetes. Because of the longer duration of their disease, many may have either peripheral or autonomic neuropathy. Clients with autonomic neuropathy generally have decreased physical work capacity due to decreased maximal heart rate and an increased resting heart rate. They easily fatigue at low work levels. In addition, older adults have an increased risk for hypotension following strenuous exercise, especially if they are deconditioned. Moreover, these clients are at increased risk for dehydration and electrolyte disturbances during exercise, particularly in warm environments. They are also more likely to experience silent ischemia. Individuals who take beta-blocking medications may not detect symptoms of hypoglycemia because these medications often mask the symptoms.

Exercise should be approached cautiously in older adults with complications of diabetes. Avoid activities that involve rapid changes in body position or elicit significant changes in heart rate or blood pressure. Clients with peripheral neuropathy may be more predisposed to traumatic injuries of the ankles and feet and to ulcerations on the lower extremities. Significant lower-limb injury can occur without their knowing it. Activities such as swimming or aquatic exercise, cycling (outdoor, stationary, or recumbent), and low-impact or chair exercise that do not stress the ankles and feet are recommended. In addition, loss of sensitivity to the lower extremities because of neuropathy can cause greater susceptibility to overstretching of muscles and connective tissue.

Clients with peripheral neuropathy may not be able to feel their pulse with their fingertips; therefore, other methods of monitoring exercise intensity should be employed. In lieu of these special medical conditions, exercise is indicated in older adults or persons with disease-related complications and can provide significant benefit.

GROUP EXERCISE CONSIDERATIONS

Many older adults are participating in exercise programs offered by local Parks and Recreation Departments, the YMCA, and facilities that offer the SilverSneakers Group Exercise Programs. The following are considerations to take into account when working with older adults in a group-exercise class setting.

When using a chair to assist with balance or when performing chair-based exercise, a straight-back, armless, steel gauge chair with a noncontoured seat to ensure proper posture and stability is recommended. Correct seated posture is forward in the chair without back support, chest up, and eyes forward.

Water containers and resistance tools can be placed under the chair for easy access and to allow participants to move safely around the chair.

It is recommended to cue participants a minimum of three times for hydration, posture, breathing, and perceived exertion. The intensity of the exercise should be rated at 5 to 8 on a 1 to 10 RPE chart.

The SilverSneakers Fitness Program follows the recommendations from the "Physical Activity and Public Health in Older Adults: Recommendation from the ACSM and the American Heart Association 2007" (Nelson et al. 2007). A recommended condition-specific class format includes:

Warm-up/stretch	5–10 min
Moderate cardio	15–20 min
Resistance work	5–10 min
Cool-down/stretch/relaxation	5 min
Total time	**30–45 min**

Group-exercise classes and personal training sessions should be taught on nonconsecutive days. Time periods most convenient for older adults are mornings and early afternoons. Classes should be taught in an area appropriate for group-exercise instruction. The SilverSneakers Fitness Program recommends 16 square feet of space per person for group-exercise classes and 3 feet between weight equipment for safety. Participants should be instructed to bring water, dress in comfortable clothing, and wear shoes with good lateral support and shock absorption qualities.

Exercise programming for older adults with diabetes should follow the physical activity recommendations listed for people with T1DM and T2DM. Special attention should be given to older adults with foot neuropathies and sight and/or balance considerations. When working in a group setting with older adults, any exercise or movement that you think might be too risky for the participants should be avoided.

In addition to the warning signs of hypoglycemia, be cognizant of any pain, swelling, muscle weakness, discoloration, disorientation, slurred speech, numbness, or profuse sweating that your participants may experience. Do not prescribe medical treatment, but encourage participants to seek the advice of their physician for any problem that occurs during class or lasts longer than two to three days.

Any injury, however slight, needs attention and written documentation. Review and practice your site's emergency plan and know the location address (Healthways 2008).

FOOT CARE FOR THE PHYSICALLY ACTIVE

Good foot care will allow an individual with diabetes to continue to exercise for years and years. Foot problems are a major complication of diabetes and can be a barrier to exercise participation. High blood glucose damages nerves and blood vessels, causing poor circulation and loss of sensation in the lower extremities and feet. These conditions make the foot vulnerable to serious injury. Diabetes can cause foot problems that if not caught early or cared for properly can result in serious problems and even require amputation.

Diabetes can affect the feet in two ways: nerve damage and blood vessel disease. Nerve damage, or neuropathy, can result from many years of high blood glucose levels. Nerve damage results in tingling, numbness, and pain in the hands and feet and can cause loss of feeling and difficulty with balance. Loss of feeling makes it difficult to feel blisters forming during exercise. In addition, less sweating and more dryness of the feet can occur, making the skin more susceptible to cracking and infection.

Lack of feeling and sensitivity in the lower extremities make it more difficult to acknowledge stretching limitations, and muscles and connective tissue can be overstretched easily. Sometimes nerve damage can cause muscle weakness and shortening of the tendons of the feet. These problems can change the contour of the feet, making it difficult to find appropriate footwear or even walk.

Diabetes can also affect the lower extremities through the development of blood vessel disease. High levels of blood glucose can damage blood vessels, resulting in diminished blood flow. Reduced blood flow results from the vessels' increased rigidity or from the build-up of plaque in the walls of vessels. Reduced blood flow interferes with the body's ability to heal an injury or fight infection.

Advise your clients to take care of their feet by following these recommendations:

- Check feet daily, especially after exercise. Note hot spots, blisters, cuts, sores, bunions, and calluses and treat them immediately.
- Engage in appropriate forms of exercise: non-weight-bearing activities such as cycling, swimming, or chair exercise may be better choices for the client with poor circulation or neuropathy in the lower extremities.
- Watch for these common foot problems: ingrown toenails, blisters, plantar warts, athlete's foot, calluses, corns, bunions, and hammer toes.
- Wear two pairs of socks or reinforced sport socks to provide extra cushioning and to avoid blisters and calluses. Cotton or wool-blend socks are best. Avoid nylon socks or stockings. Never wear shoes without socks.
- Select a comfortable and well-fitting shoe appropriate for the activity.
- Help decrease the pressure that many activities exert on the bottom of the foot by wearing special shoe inserts or insoles.
- Keep toenails trimmed and cut straight across.
- Apply a light dusting of cornstarch between the toes to help absorb excessive perspiration.
- Keep feet clean, but avoid drying soaps, excessive soaking, and extreme water temperatures. Dry feet well, especially between toes.
- Avoid activities such as basketball, tennis, hiking, and jogging if foot problems occur because they cause added stress to the feet.
- Use moisturizing skin lotion or cream on feet daily except between the toes.
- See a doctor promptly if any sign of foot injury occurs.

STUDY QUESTIONS

Complete the following questions. The answer key is on page 122.

1. Case Study: You are a high school tennis coach. One of your players has been just been diagnosed with type 1 diabetes. What is the first thing that you want to her to do:
    a. count carbohydrates before and during exercise
    b. snack immediately following practice
    c. check blood glucose levels before, during, and after practice
    d. reduce total daily insulin dose

    Is she at greater risk for hyperglycemia or hypoglycemia? What are the signs and symptoms that you will be looking for to prevent this risk?

2. Case Study: You are a group fitness teacher. Occasionally, a middle aged overweight woman attends your cycling class. You notice that she checks her blood glucose levels before and after class and she often looks frustrated. She misses a week of class, when you see her in gym one day, how might you motivate her to attend your class?

3. Case Study: Monica is 32 years old and has gestational diabetes. This is her second pregnancy and she had GDM during her first pregnancy. During her first pregnancy she did not exercise because she had previously been sedentary. She tests her blood glucose regularly and is meeting the blood glucose goal that she has set with her physician. She does not have any other health concerns and her pregnancy is proceeding well. In the past year, Monica has begun a regular program of walking 45 minutes four times per week. Now, she is going to start taking fitness classes with you (aerobics, strength training, and yoga). Is it safe for Monica to attend your fitness classes? Why or why not? What are the warning signs for exercise termination that are important for you to bring to Monica's attention?

4. Case Study: Eleanor is 72 years old, has type 2 diabetes, takes oral medications and insulin, she has peripheral neuropathy in her hands and feet and has fallen recently. She comes to you for advice regarding an exercise program that will help her to build strength and prevent another fall. What type of program would you recommend for her? How would you gauge the intensity of her workouts?

5. Case Study: Mike is an experienced cyclist going for a 3-hour ride; this is his longest ride of the season and it is a hot day. His glucose level prior to exercise is 179 mg/dl. He eats a small breakfast, reduces his insulin basal rate by 10% and the starts his ride. During exercise he checks his glucose level and it has dropped to 120 mg/dl after 1½ hours, at 2½ hours it is 80 mg/dl. When he returns home, his glucose level is 64 mg/dl. He felt hot and fatigued during the ride; the last 30 minutes of the ride were pretty tough. During the ride he sipped on water and has two sports gels. What are your recommendations for Mike to improve his performance on his next ride?

8 | PROFESSIONAL RESPONSIBILITIES

This chapter outlines your responsibilities as a professional fitness practitioner. It is not meant to be comprehensive but is a reminder of the responsibilities of a health fitness professional working with clients with diabetes. Professional responsibilities include information on health screening, medical clearance, fitness assessment, monitoring exercise, responding to acute diabetes complications, recordkeeping, terminating exercise, contraindications for exercise, risk management, emergency procedures, and physician referral.

HEALTH SCREENING FOR PHYSICAL ACTIVITY

Health screening is a crucial first step in maintaining the safety and effectiveness of any exercise program. Health screening has several purposes: (1) identifying health conditions and risk factors that put your client at risk when participating in an exercise program or may necessitate referral to a healthcare professional; (2) assisting in the design of an appropriate exercise program; (3) identifying possible contraindicated activities; (4) fulfilling legal and insurance requirements for you or your facility; and (5) encouraging and maintaining communication with the client's healthcare provider.

The Physical Activity Readiness Questionnaire (PAR-Q) and the AHA/ACSM Health/Fitness Facility Participation Screening Questionnaire have been recommended as a minimal standard for entry into low- to moderate-intensity exercise programs (ACSM 2010). More detailed medical/healthy history forms may be appropriate for clients with a chronic disease, such as diabetes, or disabilities, such as neuropathies related to diabetes.

A health screening process is a valuable tool to assist the fitness practitioner to safely and appropriately individualize the client's exercise program. Information on the form should be referred to often and updated every year or when a new condition arises. (A copy of the PAR-Q is located in the appendix.)

In addition to the general medical health screening form, the following questions specific to the client's condition may be helpful in designing a safe and effective exercise program.

71

1. **Do you routinely check blood glucose?**

   Habitual self-monitoring of blood glucose (SMBG) and measurement of gly-cosylated hemoglobin indicates an awareness of glycemic control. Exercise is riskier for individuals who do not monitor blood glucose and for those who do not have stable blood glucose throughout the day.

2. **Do you take insulin?**

   If yes, is the insulin fast-acting or slow-acting or both? Do you use an insulin pump or injections?

   People who take insulin are more prone to hypoglycemic reactions. In addition, the time release of the insulin is important in scheduling physical activity. People who use insulin pumps will have greater ability to adjust insulinization surrounding exercise by reducing their basal insulin rate.

3. **Do you take oral medications? What types?**

   Sulfonylureas and meglitinides carry hypoglycemic risks.

4. **Do you test your blood glucose surrounding exercise?**

   Encourage clients to check their blood sugar before and after exercise to avoid hyperglycemic or hypoglycemic reactions. If their exercise sessions last longer than 60 to 90 minutes, encourage them to check during exercise as well. This is of particular importance when beginning the exercise program or changing training parameters.

5. **Have you ever had a hypoglycemic or hyperglycemic reaction? If so, what happened and how did you feel?**

   This will help identify clients who are more prone to reactions and to recognize how the reaction presents in that particular client. Some of your clients may experience hypoglycemia unawareness. This means that they will rely on you to notice changes in their behaviors or personality that may indicate hypoglycemia. Your clients must be able to recognize early hypoglycemia warning signs, know how to treat hypoglycemia, and wear a medic-alert bracelet indicating diabetic status in order to exercise safely (Lisle and Trojian 2006). Clients who participate in vigorous exercise or travel for exercise should carry a glucagon shot for emergency hypoglycemic events.

6. **How do you treat your hypoglycemia?**

   Knowledge of the individual's treatment plan will help you to understand what works best for that person and is helpful in avoiding over- or under-treating the symptoms. Remember the 15–50 rule: 15 grams of carbohydrate should raise blood glucose levels 50 points in 15 minutes. When an individual experiences hypoglycemia, he or she may want to eat much more than this. Gently remind clients that they only need 15 grams of carbohydrate to return their glucose levels to normal. Once glucose has normalized, a small, balanced snack containing carbohydrate, protein, and fat will assist in maintaining blood glucose level.

7. **Have you been diagnosed as having diabetic retinopathy or neuropathy in your legs or feet?**

   If yes, does this affect your ability to walk or perform weight-bearing exercises?

Remember that the health screening process should always be supported by careful monitoring and observation during the exercise session.

Medical Clearance

If indicated by the PAR-Q or the health screening instrument, the client should be referred to his or her healthcare provider for medical clearance. It is strongly advised that clients with special medical conditions, identified as "at risk," or who exhibit symptoms during an exercise bout, obtain a medical clearance from their physician prior to the start of any exercise program.

The ACSM recommends a thorough medical exam before beginning an exercise program for individuals with known cardiovascular, pulmonary, and metabolic disease and has recommended criteria for situations that warrant a physician's release prior to exercise (ACSM 2010). Remember, however, that you reserve the right to require any participant, upon reviewing his or her medical history form, to provide a physician's release prior to admittance into an exercise program. You also reserve the right to screen individuals from your program who are deemed medically inappropriate.

It is important that any physician-signed release containing specific recommendations, modifications, or restrictions be fully respected and adhered to by the fitness practitioner. It is sound practice to have the physician establish a blood glucose upper and lower limit.

Medications

The health history form should identify any prescription or over-the-counter medications your client is taking. Some medications influence the heart's response to exercise and your client's exercise tolerance. The most feasible way to identify a medication's effect on heart rate and blood pressure response is to identify the major category of the drug and refer to a medication list like the one found in *ACSM's Guidelines for Exercise Testing and Prescription* (2010). The *Physician's Desk Reference* (PDR) is an excellent reference text for more detailed information about prescription medications and can be accessed at www.pdrhealth.com. Information regarding the primary medications prescribed for diabetes is found later in this chapter.

A client's response to medication is affected by the dose, when the medication was taken, and the individual's tolerance of the drug. It is not uncommon for people with a chronic disease or elderly people to take multiple medications, and drug interactions can occur. In general, medications used in the treatment of diabetes do not affect heart rate, blood pressure, or exercise tolerance. Other categories of medications, such as beta blockers and calcium channel blockers, will most likely affect the function of the heart and circulatory system, as will decongestants used for the common cold and bronchodilators used for asthma and other chronic obstructive pulmonary diseases (COPD). Be aware that beta blockers and other medications can interfere with the ability to discern hypoglycemic symptoms (ACSM 2010). Diet pills, caffeine, and nicotine all have stimulant properties and can increase heart rate (HR) and blood pressure (BP).

Remember that a client's response to any medication will be affected by the dose, the time the medication was taken, and the individual's tolerance of the drug. If you have any questions regarding the client's health history, medical status, medication, or physician's release, contact the physician directly.

The two primary classifications of drugs prescribed in the treatment of diabetes are insulin and oral agents. If you have any questions regarding your client's medications, side effects, or drug interactions, contact the client's physician or healthcare provider.

Insulin. Insulin always is used in the treatment of Type 1 DM and LADA, and 50% to 60% of people with Type 2 DM take insulin. Exogenous insulin is taken through injections or infused through a pump. There are four categories of insulin, and each insulin type has a general pattern of when the insulin will onset or become active, when it will peak, and how long it will continue to be active.

Insulin Type	Brand/Generic Name	Onset	Peak	Duration
Rapid acting	Humalog/insulin lispro, Novolog/insulin aspart, Apidra/insulin glusine	10–30 minutes	½–2 hours	1–4 hours
Short acting	Humulin R, Novolin R/regular insulin	½–1 hour	1½–3 hours	4–6 hours
Intermediate acting	Humulin N, Novolin N/NPH	1–3 hours	4–12 hours	18–24 hours
Long acting	Levemir/insulin detemir, Lantus/insulin glargine	2–4	None	16–24 hours

(Diabetes Forecast 2009)

Generally, rapid- or short-acting insulin is taken with meals and long-acting insulin is taken once or twice a day to provide "background" insulin. Individuals who use a pump have a basal rate of rapid insulin to provide "background" insulin, and they use boluses of rapid-acting insulin with meals. Adjustments can be made in the dose and the timing of the dose relative to exercise. Your client may also take an insulin that is a combination of rapid- or short-acting insulin with an intermediate-acting insulin. These insulins are less common.

Glucagon. Glucagon is a medication that is prescribed to people who are at risk for hypoglycemia, primarily those who use insulin. Glucagon is a hormone that increases blood glucose level. Glucagon is injected to increase blood glucose level quickly during a hypoglycemic event if the individual has lost consciousness. Glucagon stimulates hepatic glucose production and increases blood glucose within 10 to 15 minutes. All athletes should carry a glucagon shot, especially when traveling. Coaches and teammates should be familiar with glucagon and its use. When an athlete has participated in exhaustive exercise, hepatic glycogen stores may be low or depleted, in which case the glucagon shot would be ineffective (Lisle and Trojian 2006).

Oral Agents. Oral agents are used for the treatment of T2DM and GMD only. Most oral hypoglycemic agents are contraindicated during pregnancy; however, glyburide may be used. Oral agents may be used by themselves or in combination with each other or insulin. There are currently six classes of oral agents, with many new drugs rapidly entering the market and expanding the pharmaceutical options for lowering blood sugar. Available now are sulfonylureas, meglitinides, biguanides, alpha-glucosidase inhibitors, dipeptyl peptidase-4 inhibitors, and thiazolidinediones. In addition to the medications listed on the next page, there are combination pills that combine two of the medications below.

ORAL AGENTS USED FOR THE TREATMENT OF T2DM AND GDM

Medication Class	Medication Brand Name	Medication Generic Name	How It Works	Cautions
Alpha-glucosidase inhibitors	Precose Glyset	acarbose miglitol	Slows the digestion of carbohydrate	
Biguanides	Glucophage Glucophage XR, Glumetza and Riomet (liquid)	metformin	Decreases hepatic glucose production and increases muscle insulin sensitivity	
Dipeptyl peptidase-4 inhibitors	Januvia	sitagliptin	Increases insulin release after meals and reduces hepatic glucose production	
Meglitinides	Prandin Starlix	repaglinide nateglinide	Increases insulin output from the pancreas	May cause hypoglycemic reaction, although less of a risk compared with sulfonylureas
Sulfonylureas	Amaryl Glucotrol, Glucotrol X Glynase, PrexTab Diabinese	glimepiride glipizide glyburide chlorpropamide	Increases insulin output from the pancreas	May cause hypoglycemic reaction
Thiazolidinediones (TZD)	Actos Avandia	pioglitazone rosiglitazone	Decreases insulin resistance in the liver and muscles	

(Diabetes Forecast 2009)

Fitness Evaluations

Fitness evaluations are an integral part of the health screening process. They are used to assess parameters of fitness, assign beginning workloads, and serve as a baseline for future comparisons. Standard resting assessments include height, weight, resting heart rate, and resting blood pressure. Standard field tests for flexibility, muscle strength, muscle endurance, submaximal cardiovascular endurance, and body composition may be administered. Established field assessments are easily administered and are reliable methods to determine initial fitness levels and the client's exercise tolerance and limiting symptoms, as well as to monitor changes in fitness resulting from the exercise program. During the cardiovascular assessment, it is helpful to have the client note any unusual muscle or joint discomfort, pain, fatigue, or hypoglycemic response.

A client's aerobic exercise tolerance can be evaluated with a simple walking or bench-step test. Walking assessments that can be administered easily include the Rockport walk test, one-mile test, and the six- or twelve-minute walk test. Bench-step assessments include the Masters, Kasch, Getchell, and Harvard bench-step test. Treadmills and cycle ergometers can also be used in the initial or follow-up fitness testing. Exercise testing is crucial for your clients with diabetes who also exhibit signs and symptoms of the risks for cardiovascular disease (ACSM 2010). Signs and symptoms of cardiovascular disease include pain, discomfort in the chest, neck, or jaw, shortness of breath at rest or with mild exertion, dizziness or syncope, swollen ankles, palpitations or tachycardia, intermittent claudication, heart murmur, and unusual fatigue with usual activities. Risk factors for cardiovascular disease include age (>45 years for men, >55 years for women), family history, sedentary lifestyle, cigarette smoking, obesity, hypertension, dyslipidemia, pre-diabetes, and diabetes.

Clients may have clinical laboratory tests performed by their physician, including a resting ECG, lipid panel, hemoglobin A1C, and graded exercise test (stress test). Any information on the results of clinical assessments will assist you in designing the most effective program.

MONITORING EXERCISE

Several effective methods are used to monitor exercise. Minimum routine monitoring should include heart rate and perceived exertion. In clients with known cardiovascular disease, blood pressure should be monitored.

Heart Rate

Encourage clients to learn to palpate and count their own heart rate (HR) or use a heart rate monitor. Clients who have lost sensation in their finger pads may be unable to palpate their pulse, and a heart rate monitor may be indicated. If a client has difficulty finding the pulse at the carotid or radial artery, try the temporal artery. A target heart rate chart can be used to determine a target heart rate range. If the client is on heart-rate-alternating medications, such as a beta blocker, an alternative method for monitoring exercise should be used.

Perceived Exertion

The BORG Rating of Perceived Exertion (RPE) scale is an acceptable way to monitor exercise intensity and tolerance. This method works well when used in conjunction with HR monitoring. This is the preferred method for clients on HR-altering medication, clients who have pain-limiting symptoms, older clients, and clients unable to palpate their pulse rate.

RPE is recommended for clients with exertional angina, claudication, or who are extremely deconditioned. The 6–20 BORG scale and the 1–10 scale are located in the appendix. The RPE should be compatible with the client's physical appearance and rated between 11 and 16 on the 6–20 scale and between 5 and 8 on the 1–10 scale.

PVD Scale

Designed for use with clients who have peripheral vascular disease (PVD), the PVD scale is useful for clients with diabetes who experience lower-extremity pain due to autonomic or peripheral neuropathy or claudication. Claudication caused by peripheral vascular disease can be a long-term effect of diabetes. Claudication can cause pain or discomfort in the lower extremities during weight-bearing physical activity.

Talk Test

The talk test is a practical method that clients can use to help monitor exercise intensity. A client should be able to carry on a conversation with another person during exercise. If this is not possible, reduce the workload. The talk test is a particularly practical method to use with clients who are limited by shortness of breath or wheezing.

Physical Symptoms of Overwork

Practitioners, as well as clients, should be taught to observe physical signs or symptoms that indicate overwork or insulin reactions. Signs of overwork include abnormal musculoskeletal pain or discomfort, an elevated heart rate that is above what is normal for the client, red face, abnormal shortness of breath, excessive perspiration, abnormal fatigue, chest pains or palpitations, or a facial expression or body posture that indicates discomfort. In addition, clients should be instructed not to exercise during an acute illness, when fatigued, or when under excessive stress. Clients should be taught to identify inappropriate responses to exercise and to report their occurrence.

RESPONDING TO ACUTE DIABETES COMPLICATIONS

Because exercise has an insulin-like effect, exercise-induced hypoglycemia is the most common acute complication your clients with diabetes will experience during or after exercise. Hyperglycemia rarely occurs as a direct result of exercise; however, an individual may, for various reasons, have significant hyperglycemia while working with you. It is important to know the signs and symptoms of hypoglycemia and hyperglycemia and how to respond.

Hypoglycemia

Hypoglycemia, or low blood sugar, occurs quickly and symptoms onset rapidly. Biological hypoglycemia is considered to be 50 mg/dl or less. Severe symptoms generally occur when the blood glucose level drops below 40 mg/dl, although this is highly individual. When treated, symptoms disappear quickly, usually in 10 to 15 minutes. Symptoms of hypoglycemia include sudden hunger, dizziness, shakiness, headache, butterflies in the stomach, sweatiness, irritability, fatigue, weakness, sensitivity to light, tingling on tongue, and blurred vision. Several factors are related to the development of hypoglycemic reactions:

- Exercise increases the uptake of glucose into cells, thereby reducing blood glucose level.
- Too much insulin inhibits glucagon and blocks fatty acid use (increasing glucose uptake by cells).
- Too little carbohydrate for the exercise intensity or duration or for the insulinization.
- Skipping or delaying meals can predispose the individual to hypoglycemia.

It is the fitness practitioner's responsibility to proceed accordingly with the following actions when a hypoglycemic reaction occurs or is suspected:

1. Stop, discontinue exercise, and check blood glucose if a meter is available.
2. Have the client ingest 15 grams of carbohydrate such as 4 ounces orange juice, 1 Fig Newton, 8 ounces regular soda, or 5 Lifesavers. Avoid foods that also contain fat; fat slows the absorption of carbohydrate.
3. Recheck blood glucose in 15 minutes. If within normal ranges and when symptoms disappear, client may resume exercise.
4. Resume activity only when blood glucose levels are appropriate.
5. Client should ingest more substantial CHOs in addition to some protein after exercise.
6. If the condition continues on a regular basis, refer the client to his or her physician.

Hyperglycemia

Hyperglycemia, or high blood sugar, has a slow onset. Symptoms of hyperglycemia include increased thirst and urination, headache, nausea, vomiting, and drowsiness. Several factors can contribute to hyperglycemia:

- Too much food intake relative to insulin availability and action or exercise intensity and duration.
- Too little insulin prevents enough glucose from entering the cells.
- Illness, stress, or infection may increase blood sugar.

In case of symptomatic hyperglycemia, the fitness practitioner's responsibilities are:

1. Have the client check his or her blood glucose levels.
2. Have the client take insulin or oral medication if it was not taken at the scheduled time.
3. Have the client consume fluids to prevent dehydration.
4. If blood glucose levels are more than 250 mg/dl, encourage your client to check his or her urine for ketones. Do not exercise when blood glucose is more than 300 mg/dl, regardless of the presence of ketones.
5. Contact the physician or healthcare provider.
6. Delay exercise until blood glucose is controlled.

Hyperglycemia is not likely to occur as a result of exercise because exercise facilitates the utilization of insulin and glucose. However, if a client starts exercising with inadequate insulin and an elevated glucose level, their glucose will likely continue to rise during exercise. In a hypoinsulinemic state, the body begins to burn fat and protein for energy because glucose is not available. The by-product of fat and protein metabolism is ketones. As ketones in the blood rise, the blood becomes more acidic, leading to a dangerous condition called ketoacidosis. Symptoms of ketoacidosis include stomach pain, dehydration, fruity breath, nausea, vomiting, and drowsiness. A diabetic coma can occur when ketoacidosis is present. This is a life-threatening situation and medical treatment should be immediate.

RECORDKEEPING

Recordkeeping is important to demonstrate objective improvement to the client, practitioner, and healthcare provider and to assist in guiding the progression of exercise. It is also helpful in determining normal and abnormal responses to exercise training. This is particularly true for heart rate and blood pressure responses at rest and during exercise, as well as blood glucose fluctuations that may occur during or after exercise. If the client were to have any problem during or after exercise, documentation of exercise progression and tolerance would be important. Any changes in medication or physician recommendations should be noted. Copies of the patient's daily logs, including diet, blood glucose levels, and exercise intensity and duration are invaluable.

The procedures for documentation may vary, depending on the exercise facility and client status. For example, the documentation in a medically based diabetes program may be much more extensive than that done in a community-based fitness program or in a one-on-one training session. Be sure to note any abnormal responses to exercise that occur during a session. This documentation can be kept on the client's daily workout log for the individual training day. It should be noted that a client whose function is not maintained or does not improve with adequate adherence to appropriate exercise requires physician evaluation.

CRITERIA FOR TERMINATION OF EXERCISE

The following are unhealthy responses to exercise and signs of overexertion that indicate termination of the exercise:

- Excessive fatigue
- Signs or symptoms of hypoglycemia or hyperglycemia
- Abnormal muscle or joint discomfort or pain
- Inappropriate shortness of breath (SOB)
- Dizziness, lightheadedness, nausea, confusion
- Excessive tachycardia or inappropriate bradycardia
- Leg pain, cramping
- Failure to increase HR with increased workload
- Onset of angina with exercise
- Client requests to stop the exercise

CONTRAINDICATIONS FOR EXERCISE

The following situations contraindicate exercise:

- Scuba diving, parachute jumping, rock climbing, and other high-risk sports should only be done with specific training because it would be difficult to treat an insulin reaction during these sports. Highly skilled training is necessary. Training and assistance for these individuals can be found through the International Diabetes Athletes Association. Participation in these sports is possible with the appropriate training and planning.
- People with proliferating diabetic retinopathy should refrain from sudden anaerobic physical exertion, including weight training. Diabetic retinopathy is a disorder in which small blood vessels nourishing the retina

weaken and break down. These tiny vessels can hemorrhage with sudden increased pressure. These clients should avoid weightlifting, bodybuilding, and power lifting because these activities are associated with increased blood pressure and risk of retinal hemorrhage. In fact, it has been recommended that diabetics suffering from diabetic retinopathy not perform cardiopulmonary resuscitation. Any activity that elevates the systolic blood pressure above 180–200 mmHg for substantial periods of time should be avoided.

- Neuropathy in the lower extremities can be aggravated by pounding or impact activities. Therefore, impact and weight-bearing exercise such as running or hiking should be avoided if neuropathy is present. Bicycling, swimming, and chair exercise should be encouraged.
- If blood sugar is above 250, urine should be tested for ketones prior to exercise.
- If ketones are present, exercise is contraindicated. If blood glucose is more than 300 mg/dl, regardless of ketones, exercise is contraindicated.
- Dehydration.
- Signs and symptoms of hypoglycemia prior to exercise.

RISK MANAGEMENT

Every fitness professional must have a risk-management plan to ensure the safety and effectiveness of the exercise program. A basic risk-management plan includes the following: (1) identification of risk areas; (2) evaluation of specific risks in each area; (3) selection of appropriate treatment for each risk; (4) implementation of a risk-management system; and (5) evaluation of success. In addition, risk management includes establishing contact with your client's healthcare team, knowing when to refer your client to his or her physician, and knowing and following emergency procedures.

Emergency Procedures

It is important to know emergency medical procedures and have a system in place for responding to a medical emergency. An emergency plan must be devised for every training situation. In a medical emergency situation, the victim needs medical help immediately. Act quickly and insist on prompt medical attention, even if the person resists. First, call an emergency rescue service, 911, or immediately take the client to a hospital emergency department. While waiting for emergency medical services to arrive, keep the person quiet, in a half-sitting position, and try to relieve his or her anxiety. Loosen tight-fitting clothing and maintain an even body temperature. Do not lift the person or give him or her food or drink. Treat with CHO only if exhibiting symptoms of hypoglycemia.

Establishing Physician Contact

Establishing and developing contact and rapport with the medical community will greatly enhance your ability to provide for your clients with diabetes. There are benefits in developing relationships between the physician and fitness practitioner for the client, as well as for the involved professionals. It ensures a safe program for clients and establishes credibility with physicians and healthcare providers. It builds a potential referral system between the fitness practitioner and the medical community. It also is an excellent way to obtain educational information for the fitness trainer as well as the physician.

Client Privacy

It is the fitness professional's responsibility to comply with the federal government's 2004 Privacy Act by doing the following:

- When a client begins to discuss personal health issues, escort the client to a private setting, if possible, away from the hearing range of others.
- If you learn that a client is planning to be absent from a group-exercise class due to a health-related issue (illness, surgery, hospitalization):
  - Ask the client what, if anything, you can share with others if you are asked about the client's absence.
  - If a client's absence from class is obvious to others, acknowledge the absence without providing any personal details.
- When talking about the benefits of exercise or coaching for modifications to exercises specific to certain conditions, speak generally without referring to any specific class member.

Immediate Physician Referral

If your client with diabetes experiences any of the following symptoms during or following an exercise session, he or she should ***stop*** exercising ***immediately*** and call his or her physician ***today:***

- Unstable blood glucose
- Onset of angina or chest pain with exercise
- Severe pain from injury
- Numbness or tingling in an arm or leg
- Signs of progressive fatigue, severe thirst, frequent urination, nausea, or vomiting

If symptoms do not subside with rest or sugar, or if there is loss of consciousness, activate EMS (Emergency Medical Response System).

STUDY QUESTIONS

Complete the following questions. The answer key is on page 123.

1. Your client shows signs of hypoglycemia during your training session. Outline the steps you would take.

2. List three factors that can contribute to hyperglycemia.

3. List five to six strategies to avoid hypoglycemia during exercise.

4. When should exercise be terminated?

APPENDIX: MONITORING EXERCISE

The Physical Activity Readiness Questionnaire (PAR-Q) has been recommended as a minimal standard for entry into low- to moderate-intensity exercise programs. The Rating of Perceived Exertion scale and the PVD Scale are tools to assist in monitoring tolerance of exercise by the client. The Exercise Log can be used by clients to monitor their their glucose response surrounding exercise.

Physical Activity
Readiness
Questionnaire
PAR-Q

PAR-Q & YOU

(A Questionnaire for People Ages 15 to 69)

Regular physical activity is fun and healthy. More people are becoming increasingly active every day. Being active is very safe for most people. However, some people should check with their doctor before they increase their physical activity.

If you are planning to become more physically active, start by answering the seven questions in the box below. If you are between the ages of 15 and 69, the PAR-Q will tell you if you should check with your doctor before you start. If you are over 69 years of age and you are not used to being very active, check with your doctor.

Common sense is your best guide when you answer these questions. Please read the questions carefully and answer each one honestly. Check YES or NO.

YES	NO	
❏	❏	1. Has your doctor ever said that you have a heart condition and that you should only do physical activity recommended by a doctor?
❏	❏	2. Do you feel pain in your chest when you do physical activity?
❏	❏	3. In the past month, have you had chest pain when you were not doing physical activity?
❏	❏	4. Do you lose your balance because of dizziness or do you ever lose consciousness?
❏	❏	5. Do you have a bone or joint problem that could be made worse by a change in your physical activity?
❏	❏	6. Is your doctor currently prescribing drugs (for example, water pills) for your blood pressure or heart condition?
❏	❏	7. Do you know of *any other reason* why you should not perform physical activity?

If you answered

YES to one or more questions

Talk with your doctor BEFORE you start becoming more physically active or BEFORE you have a fitness appraisal. Tell your doctor about the PAR-Q and which questions you answered YES.

- You may be able to do any activity you want to—as long as you start slowly and buildup gradually. Or you may need to restrict your activities to those that are safe for you. Talk with your doctor about the kinds of activities you wish to participate in and follow his/her advice.
- Find out which community programs are safe and helpful for you.

NO to all questions

If you answered NO to *all* PAR-Q questions, you can be reasonably sure that you can:

- Start becoming more physically active—begin slowly and buildup gradually. That is the safest and easiest way to go.
- Take part in a fitness appraisal—this is an excellent way to determine your basic fitness so that you plan the best way for you to live actively.

Delay becoming more active:
- If you are not feeling well because of a temporary illness such as a cold or a fever—wait until you feel better.
- If you are or may be pregnant—talk with your doctor before you become more active.

Rating of Perceived Exertion (Borg Scale)

6–20 Scale		0–10 Scale	
6		0	Nothing at all
7	Very, very light	.5	Very, very weak
8		1	Very weak
9	Very light	2	Weak
10		3	Moderate
11	Fairly light	4	Somewhat strong
12		5	Strong
13	Somewhat hard	6	
14		7	Very strong
15	Hard	8	
16		9	
17	Very hard	10	Very, very strong
18			
19			
20	Very, very hard		

The rating of perceived exertion (RPE) should be compatible with the client's physical appearance. Ratings between 11 and 16 on the 6–20 scale and between 3 and 7 on the revised 1–10 scale are desirable.

PVD SCALE

0	No claudication pain
1	Initial, minimal pain
2	Moderate pain
3	Intense pain
4	Maximal pain, cannot continue

BLOOD GLUCOSE, FOOD, AND MEDICATION LOG FOR EXERCISE

NAME

Date

Time

	Blood Glucose	Food and Fluid Intake	Medications	Comments
Before exercise				
During exercise				
After exercise				

Date

Time

	Blood Glucose	Food and Fluid Intake	Medications	Comments
Before exercise				
During exercise				
After exercise				

✳ GLOSSARY

bolus. One dose of insulin.

claudication. Pain that occurs in a muscle with an inadequate blood supply, usually as a result of cardiovascular disease, that is stressed by exercise. The pain does not occur when sitting or standing, is reproducible from day to day, is more severe when walking upstairs or up a hill, and is often described as a cramp, which disappears within 1–2 minutes of finishing exercise (ACSM 2010).

endogenous. Produced within the body.

exogenous. From outside the body.

glucagon. A hormone that increases blood glucose levels, it is released from the liver when blood glucose levels drop and it may be used as an injection to quickly increase blood glucose levels during severe hypoglycemia.

glycogen. Stored glucose in the liver and muscle.

hepatic. Refers to the liver.

insulin infusion. Insulin provided through an insulin pump.

insulinization. Level of circulating insulin.

ketoacidosis. A dangerous condition of hyperglycemia resulting from a lack of circulating insulin.

neuropathy. Degradation and disease of the nervous system; a potential long-term condition of diabetes.

syncope. Fainting.

tachycardia. Increased or racing heart rate.

✳ Client Handouts

The client handouts in this section are presented in copy-ready form and may be reproduced and distributed to the clients in your training program.

- Get Ready to Exercise
- Establishing Your Independent Exercise Program
- Benefits of Exercise
- Safe Exercise Checklist
- Manage Your Blood Glucose
- Managing Your Blood Glucose Surrounding Exercise
- Hypoglycemia
- New Guidelines: Diabetes and Exercise
- Hydration
- Take Care of Your Feet
- Relaxation Techniques for Stress Management
- Tips for Healthy Living with Diabetes

GET READY TO EXERCISE

What to Wear

- Choose loose, stretchable clothing for the exercise session. A breathable fabric such as cotton or the latest synthetic material made for exercise will allow the body to ventilate and stay cool.
- Opt for a short-sleeve or sleeveless shirt rather than long sleeves or a jacket that will restrict movement and potentially cause overheating.
- Choose pants of breathable knit fabric rather than polyester or plastic "sweat" pants.
- Shorts, capri-length, and long pants are acceptable.
- Avoid wearing heavy cotton sweatsuits or sweatshirts, jeans, or tight-wasted pants for the actual exercise session.

Footwear

- A high-quality athletic shoe is recommended to promote effective and safe exercise.
- Choose a cross-trainer or running shoe with good shock absorption and support and a higher, mid-cut shoe style if support is needed for the ankle.
- Avoid flat-bottomed court shoes such as Keds and Converse.
- Invest in a new shoe if the current shoe is over a year old or has been walked in for more than 100 hours (2 hours a week for a year) for either leisure or exercise.
- Avoid dress shoes, open-toed shoes, sandals, and high-soled shoes that restrict side-to-side movement. The new Sketcher shoe promoted for shaping the legs and weight loss should not be worn.
- The shoe should fit well, be comfortable and not rub or chafe the heel, ankle, or foot.

Socks

- Choose mid-weight socks of cotton or fabric made specifically for activity that will absorb moisture and keep the feet comfortable and dry.
- Avoid synthetic fashion socks and nylons.
- Choose a sock that fits the foot and does not have seams that rub on contact points of the shoe.

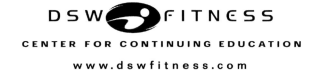

What to Bring

- A water bottle (no glass)
- A small sweat towel
- Glucose meter and lancets
- A fast-acting glucose snack: Fig Newtons, orange juice, granola bar

What and When to Eat and Drink Pre-exercise

- It is important to maintain stable blood glucose levels throughout the day and especially going into an exercise session. Follow these pre-exercise nutrition guidelines:
- Eat breakfast, lunch, dinner and snacks on your regular schedule pre-exercise. Ideally, a meal or snack should be eaten 1–3 hours before exercising.
- **Do not** skip breakfast or lunch before exercising.
- Before a late afternoon workout, eat a carbohydrate snack an hour or so before exercising, such as a banana, granola bar, crackers, yogurt, sports drink, sports chews (Cliff Shot Bloks) or sports gel (Gu).
- If your blood glucose is less than 70 mg/dl before or during exercise, stop and follow the 15-50 rule: Ingest 15 grams of carbohydrate to increase blood glucose approximately 50 points in 15 minutes.

> **Examples of 15 grams of carbohydrate**
> 4 oz fruit juice
> 8 oz sports drink
> 8 oz regular soda
> ½ banana
> 1 Fig Newton
> 3 Life Savers candies

- Eat a small snack and drink water immediately following exercise.
- Eat a meal within 2–4 hours after exercise to avoid postexercise hypoglycemia.

Hydration Guidelines

- Drink 16–24 ounces of fluid slowly in the hours before exercise plus 8 ounces immediately before the exercise session.
- Drink before you are thirsty, quenching your thirst without forcing yourself to drink.

ESTABLISHING YOUR INDEPENDENT EXERCISE PROGRAM

Consistency with your physical activity is essential in managing your blood glucose. Your independent exercise assignment is to:

- Schedule an exercise session to perform on your own or with a friend 1 time per week. Select a specific day and time for your exercise.
- Choose an activity that you enjoy. Here are several suggestions:
  - Perform the health club circuit following the protocol and exercise prescription listed on the exercise log filed at the facility.
  - Choose a group exercise class that meets the 30-minute minimum aerobic exercise criterion—aerobics, step training, spinning, aquatic aerobics
  - Complete a walk, jog, bicycle, or swim workout that meets the 30-minute minimum aerobic criterion.
- Include resistance training as part of the independent workout, but it must be in addition to the aerobic exercise.
- Remember to warm up and cool down with each exercise session.
- Match the intensity of the aerobic exercise to your intensity level during supervised circuit training.
- Monitor your RPE and exercise heart rate once during the exercise session.
- Check your blood glucose pre- and postexercise.
- Record each independent exercise session in an exercise log (see back).

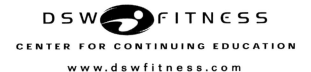

Independent Exercise Log

	BG Pre/Post	Activity MIN	HR	RPE		BG Pre/Post	Activity MIN	HR	RPE
Week 1					**Week 5**				
SUN					SUN				
MON					MON				
TUES					TUES				
WED					WED				
THU					THU				
FRI					FRI				
SAT					SAT				
Week 2					**Week 6**				
SUN					SUN				
MON					MON				
TUES					TUES				
WED					WED				
THU					THU				
FRI					FRI				
SAT					SAT				
Week 3					**Week 7**				
SUN					SUN				
MON					MON				
TUES					TUES				
WED					WED				
THU					THU				
FRI					FRI				
SAT					SAT				
Week 4					**Week 8**				
SUN					SUN				
MON					MON				
TUES					TUES				
WED					WED				
THU					THU				
FRI					FRI				
SAT					SAT				

BENEFITS OF EXERCISE

Physical activity is a key element in the prevention and management of type 2 diabetes mellitus (T2DM). A combined program of aerobic exercise and resistance training provides these specific benefits for people with diabetes:

- Lowers blood glucose levels and improves the body's ability to use glucose.
- Reduces the amount of insulin or hypoglycemic medication needed to control diabetes.
- Helps to reverse the insulin resistance that is associated with excess body fat and is implicated in the etiology of T2DM.
- Delays or prevents the development of atherosclerosis and risk factors related to heart disease, including blood pressure and elevated lipids, which are major threats to people with diabetes.
- Improves weight loss and body fat loss when combined with a reduction in caloric intake.
- Increases circulation to all parts of the body, therefore lessening the risk for the long-term complication of impaired circulation.
- Prevents the development of type 2 diabetes mellitus.
- Reduces depression.
- Reduces stress.
- Assists in managing diabetes and living a normal life.

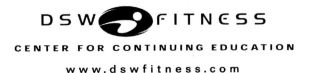

✓ SAFE EXERCISE CHECKLIST

Safety when exercising is always a priority. The following checklist will help to ensure safe and effective exercise and blood sugar management.

- ☐ Obtain a medical release from your physician or healthcare provider prior to beginning an exercise program.
- ☐ Progress through your exercise program gradually.
- ☐ Be consistent with your exercise. Try to exercise at the same time of day and at similar intensities, durations, and frequencies. Consistency results in less fluctuation in blood sugar.
- ☐ Check your blood glucose level prior to engaging in exercise. Do not initiate exercise if blood glucose levels are less than 100 mg/dl or greater than 300 mg/dl or greater than 250 mg/dl if ketones are present.
- ☐ Check your blood glucose more frequently when you start a new exercise program or when you change your exercise program.
- ☐ Monitor and record your blood glucose before, during, and after exercise. In addition, the type, duration, and intensity of exercise should be logged.
- ☐ Keep a log of food consumed before and after exercise, especially if food intake varies dramatically.
- ☐ Carry a carbohydrate-rich snack with you during exercise.
- ☐ Avoid exercise that results in dramatic increases in blood pressure.
- ☐ Wear identification that states you have diabetes.
- ☐ Wear well-fitting, supportive shoes.

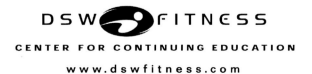

MANAGE YOUR BLOOD GLUCOSE

The **number-one goal** of diabetes treatment is to manage blood sugar levels. Some of the ways this can be done include:

- Eat a healthy diet.
- Get regular physical activity.
- Take medicine as advised by your physician.
- Test blood glucose regularly.
- Measure hemoglobin A1C every 3–6 months.
- Discuss barriers to achieving blood glucose goals with your physician.

Blood Glucose Recommendations

Discuss blood glucose targets with your diabetes management team. Two professional entities give recommendations for blood glucose levels:

✓ The **American Academy of Clinical Endocrinologists** (2008) recommends most people with diabetes aim for the following blood glucose goals:

Before meals:	70–110 mg/dl
2 hours after meals:	<140 mg/dl
At bedtime:	100–140 mg/dl

✓ The **American Diabetes Association** (2008) recommends the following goals:

Before meals:	70–130 mg/dl
1–2 hours after meals:	<180 mg/dl

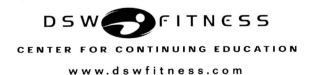

MANAGE YOUR BLOOD GLUCOSE SURROUNDING EXERCISE

Beginning a regular exercise program requires you pay attention to and manage your blood sugar surrounding exercise. Monitoring blood glucose levels pre- and postexercise will help to ensure that you consume the right amount of fuel and liquids for you activity level.

Factors that Affect Blood Glucose Surrounding Exercise

The glycemic response to a single session of exercise is dependent on several factors:

1. Blood glucose level prior to exercise
2. Intensity, duration, and type of exercise
3. Level of circulating insulin (insulinization)
4. Food and fluid intake surrounding exercise
5. Climate and stress

Manage Your Blood Glucose Surrounding Exercise

The following are possible regimen changes that can improve glycemic control. Consider each of these factors with your diabetes management team to improve your blood glucose.

- Level of insulinization surrounding exercise
- Pre-exercise meal
- Pre-exercise insulin adjustments
- During-exercise carbohydrate supplementation
- During-exercise hydration plan
- During-exercise insulin adjustments
- Postexercise carbohydrate supplementation
- Postexercise insulin adjustments

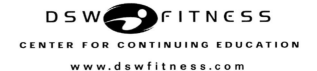

✓ HYPOGLYCEMIA

Hypoglycemia is a sudden drop in blood sugar level. It should be treated immediately.

How to Avoid Hypoglycemia

- Monitor blood glucose before, during, and after exercise.
- Consume a balanced snack before and after exercise.
- Adjust insulin dosage accordingly.
- Avoid injecting insulin into vigorously exercised muscle.
- Consume 30–75 grams carbohydrate per hour during high-intensity exercise or endurance exercise.
- Carry quick-acting sugar during exercise.

Signs of Hypoglycemia Specific to Exercise

- Abnormal gait or clicking feet when running
- Lack of balance
- Fatigue or confusion
- Chills
- Clammy
- Buzzing in ears
- Increased heart rate
- Shaky hands
- Irritability
- Reduction in power (cannot keep up with workout partners or perform at usual level)
- Heart palpitations

Treating Hypoglycemia

When blood glucose is less than 70 mg/dl or less than 100 mg/dl immediately before exercise:

1. Consume 15 grams of carbohydrate:
   - ½ banana or 1 Fig Newton
   - 8 oz sports drink or 4 oz juice
2. Check blood glucose in 15 minutes. Blood glucose levels should increase about 50 points for 15 grams of carbohydrate.
3. Repeat until glucose levels return to a normal level (70–120 mg/dl), or perhaps higher, depending on the level of insulinization (level of circulating insulin).

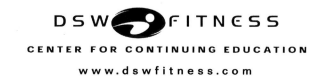

NEW GUIDELINES: DIABETES AND EXERCISE

In a Joint Position Statement, the American College of Sports Medicine (ACSM) and the American Diabetes Association (ADA) issued new exercise guidelines in 2010 for type 2 diabetes mellitus (T2DM). The new guidelines call for both aerobic and resistance training exercise and provide specific advice for those whose diabetes might limit vigorous exercise. The position statement states that:

- Exercise plays a major role in the prevention and control of insulin resistance, pre-diabetes, gestational diabetes mellitus (GDM), T2DM, and diabetes-related health complications and can assist with cardiovascular risk, mortality, and quality of life.
- Physical activity is critical for optimal health in individuals with T2DM.
- Exercise must be undertaken regularly in order to produce continued benefits.
- Both aerobic exercise and resistance training should be included in exercise programming for diabetes management.

The Guidelines for Aerobic Exercise and Resistance Training Include the Following:

Aerobic Exercise Guidelines

Frequency	3 times/week minimum; preferably 5 times/week. No more than 2 consecutive days between bouts (due to transient nature of exercise on insulin action).
Intensity	Moderate intensity. Greater health benefits can be achieved at higher intensities. Higher intensity results in improvements in overall blood glucose control more effectively than increased duration or frequency of exercise.
Duration	At least 150 minutes per week. Exercise bouts should be at least 10 minutes in duration.
Mode	Type of exercise that uses large muscle groups
Progression	Gradually for some individuals with T2DM and for those with cardiovascular, orthopedic, and other physical limitations.

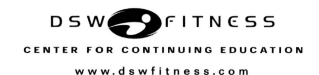

Resistance Training Guidelines

Frequency	2 times/week minimum; nonconsecutive days; progress to 3 times/week
Intensity	Initially at 50% of 1 Repetition Maximum (1RM) for 10–15 reps. Gradually increase to 75–80% of 1RM for 8–10 reps.
Duration	5–10 exercises for major muscle groups.
Mode	Strength exercise machines or free weights can be used—both have shown equivalent benefits for blood glucose control.
Progression	For greater blood glucose control, gradually increase with heavier weights first rather than adding more sets.
Sets	Start with 1 set per exercise; progress to 2–3 sets.

The ACSM and ADA recommend supervision by a qualified exercise trainer to ensure optimal blood glucose and other health benefits while minimizing the risk of injury.

To view the "Exercise and Type 2 Diabetes: American College of Sports Medicine and the American Diabetes Association: Joint Position Statement," visit http://journals.lww.com/acsm-msse/Fulltext/2010/12000/Exercise_and_Type_2_Diabetes__American_College_of.18.aspx

✓ STAY HYDRATED

People with diabetes have a greater risk of dehydration because of the increased fluid requirement of the kidneys and the urine output needed to flush excess glucose from the body if their glucose levels tend to remain above normal. Follow these steps to prevent dehydration:

- Drink plenty of fluids each day.
- To rehydrate, consume 16–24 ounces per pound of body weight.
- Monitor urine volume and color. A small amount of dark urine can be a sign of dehydration.
    - Drink cool, uncarbonated water before, during, and after exercise:
    - 20 oz or 2½ cups (600 ml) 2 hours before exercise
    - 8–16 oz (250–500 ml) 30 minutes before exercise
    - 4 oz (90–160 ml) every 15 minutes during exercise
    - As indicated by body weight and symptoms after exercise
    - Drink to satisfy thirst; don't force yourself to drink more

- Recognize the symptoms of dehydration:
    - Severe thirst
    - Dizziness
    - Tachycardia (fast heart rate)
    - Confusion
    - Headache
    - Irritability

- Weigh yourself before and after exercise — a loss of more than 2% body weight indicates dehydration.

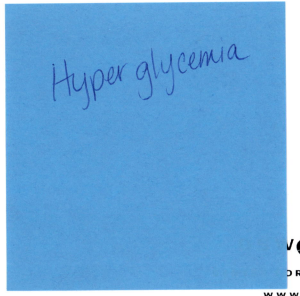

Hyperglycemia

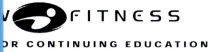

www.dswfitness.com

TAKE CARE OF YOUR FEET

Good foot care will allow you to continue to exercise and to manage foot problems. Foot problems are a major complication of diabetes and can be a barrier to exercise participation. High blood glucose damages nerves and blood vessels, causing poor circulation and loss of sensation in the lower extremities and feet. These conditions make the feet vulnerable to serious injury. Foot problems that are not caught early or cared for properly can result in serious conditions and even require amputation.

Take care of your feet by following these recommendations:

- Check feet daily, especially after exercise. Note hot spots, blisters, cuts, sores, bunions, and calluses and treat them immediately.
- Engage in appropriate forms of exercise: nonweight-bearing activities such as cycling, swimming, and chair exercise might be better choices if you have poor circulation or neuropathy in the lower extremities.
- Watch for these common foot problems: ingrown toenails, blisters, plantar warts, athlete's foot, calluses, corns, bunions, and hammer toes.
- Wear two pairs of socks or reinforced sport socks to provide extra cushioning and to avoid blisters and calluses. Cotton and wool-blend socks are best. Avoid nylon socks or stockings. Never wear shoes without socks.
- Select a comfortable and well-fitting shoe appropriate for the activity.
- Help decrease the pressure that many activities exert on the bottom of the foot by wearing special shoe inserts or insoles.
- Keep toenails trimmed and cut straight across.
- Apply a light dusting of cornstarch between the toes to help absorb excessive perspiration.
- Keep feet clean, but avoid drying soaps, excessive soaking, and extreme water temperatures. Dry feet well, especially between toes.
- Avoid activities such as basketball, tennis, hiking, and jogging if foot problems occur because these activities are stressful on the feet.
- Use moisturizing skin lotion or cream on feet daily except between the toes.
- See a doctor promptly if any sign of foot injury occurs.

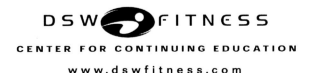

CENTER FOR CONTINUING EDUCATION

www.dswfitness.com

RELAXATION TECHNIQUES FOR STRESS MANAGEMENT

Take at least 10 to 15 minutes a day for yourself. Lie down, breathe deeply, relax completely, and be at peace with yourself. Relaxation techniques are most effectively performed in a comfortable sitting or lying position with the eyes closed and glasses removed. The relaxation space should be warm, dimly lit, and quiet. Try these relaxation techniques to find what works best for you.

Diaphragmatic Breathing

Inhale through the nose and exhale through the mouth. For diaphragmic breathing to occur, the abdomen should expand on inhalation and contract on exhalation. A hand can be placed on the abdomen to ensure this is happening. Let the chest expand and shoulders lift slightly on inhalation and then let the chest sink toward the floor and shoulders relax on exhalation. Try to roll the breath from the abdomen to the upper chest in a full wave of inhalation. Di... on technique by itself or combined with oth...

Jacobson's Progr... (Tension/Relaxati...

You must recognize how a ter... ease the tension. Contract the muscles st... ith the large muscle groups and move to t... the buttocks muscles for 5 seconds and the... en relax. The emphasis is placed on detectin... that tension. Jacobson also emphasizes the... jaw muscles. Try to "unhinge the jaw, smoot...

Autogenic Relaxa...

Autogenic means self-generated. In this technique, relaxation is brought about by concentration upon phrases of preselected words. You can focus on the heaviness of the limbs, warmth of the limbs, breathing regulation, and coolness in the forehead. For example, "slow the breathing with deep, full breaths" or "allow the feet and calves to feel heavy and sink into the floor."

Imagery

Using images is a form of mild self-hypnosis that helps take the mind off anxieties and unwanted tensions. While sitting or lying in a relaxed position, imagine "floating on a raft on a warm sunny day" or "sinking into a soft pillow or mattress."

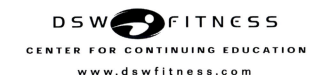

CENTER FOR CONTINUING EDUCATION

www.dswfitness.com

TIPS FOR HEALTHY LIVING WITH DIABETES

Monitor Your Blood Glucose
- Test your blood glucose. Ask your healthcare provider when to test, how often, and what your blood glucose targets are.
- Measure hemoglobin A1C every 3-6 months.
- Keep a record of your blood tests, medications, and daily activity. Review the record with your healthcare provider.

Medications
- Take your diabetes medicine as prescribed.
- Understand how your medications work and their side effects.

Eat Foods to Manage Your Blood Glucose
- See a registered dietitian to create an eating plan that is right for you.

Be Physically Active
- If you haven't been active, start slowly.
- Good activities to begin with are walking and swimming.

Maintain a Weight That Is Right for You
- Ask your healthcare provider what you should weigh and work with your registered dietitian to achieve this weight.

Prevent Complications
- Check your feet for cuts, blisters, red spots, and swelling. Call your healthcare provider right away about any sores that do not heal.
- Have an annual eye exam.
- Ask for regular blood pressure checks, cholesterol tests, and other blood fat tests.
- See your dentist at least twice a year. Tell your dentist you have diabetes.
- Have your feet, eyes, and kidneys checked at least once a year, or more often if you have problems.
- Treat low blood glucose quickly with glucose tablets or gels.
- Don't smoke. Talk to your healthcare provider about ways to quit.

Work with a Diabetes Management Team
- Learn more about diabetes and diabetes self-care. Ask your healthcare provider to suggest a registered dietitian, exercise specialist, and a diabetes educator to help you manage your diabetes.
- Write down your questions and take them with you to each visit with any member of your healthcare team.
- Seek support from family and friends or join a diabetes support group. Call your local hospital or health department to find a support group.

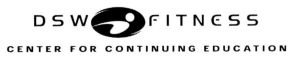

CENTER FOR CONTINUING EDUCATION

www.dswfitness.com

✳ ANSWER KEYS

Chapter 1: Introduction to Diabetes

1. True.
2. The rise in central body fatness, and sedentary lifestyle, a diet of processed foods high in calories, television watching, smoking, and low socio-economic status.
3. Non–Hispanic blacks, Mexican American, American Indian and Alaska Native, Asian, Native Hawaiian, and other Pacific Islanders.
4. Type 1.
5. The rise in central body fatness, and sedentary lifestyle, a diet of processed foods high in calories, television watching, smoking, and low socio-economic status.
6. True.

Chapter 2: Understanding Diabetes

1. Glucose if formed exogenously (externally) from food or endogenously (internally) in the liver and muscles. Following a meal, the carbohydrate in food is broken down by stomach acid and digestive enzymes into glucose. As carbohydrate is metabolized, glucose moves from the gastrointestinal tract into the bloodstream. Glucose must then move from the bloodstream in to cells to be used as energy. The liver and muscles store glucose in the form of glycogen. When additional glucose is needed, endogenous glucose production occurs. Glycogen is broken down into glucose and released in small amounts from the liver to keep blood glucose levels stable or released in larger amounts from the muscle to fuel exercise.
2. It allows glucose, from food or internal production, to pass into cells, out of the bloodstream and to be used for energy and it assists in shutting off excess internal glucose production in the liver and muscles.
3. False.
4. Type 1 is an autoimmune condition that leads to destruction of insulin producing beta cells in the pancreas; in Type 2 the pancreas makes insulin

117

however cells cannot properly utilize insulin to reduce blood glucose. As T2DM progresses, the pancreas may make insufficient insulin.

5. • Frequent urination.
   • Excessive thirst.
   • Excessive fatigue.
   • Sudden weight loss.
   • Constant or extreme hunger.
   • Blurred vision.
   • Repeated or hard to heal infections of the skin.
   • Increased gum or urinary tract infections.
   • Dry, itchy skin.
   • Tingling or loss of feeling in the hands or feet.

6. • Sedentary lifestyle.
   • Family history of diabetes in a first degree relative.
   • Overweight or obesity prior to pregnancy.
   • Over age 35.
   • Prior deliveries of large birth-weight babies (over 10 lb).
   • Repeated miscarriages or spontaneous abortions in previous pregnancies.
   • A history of glucose in the urine in a previous or current pregnancy.
   • A history of GDM.
   • Family history of diabetes.
   • Ethnicity (Hispanic, South Asian, Asian, or African descent).

7. Ketosis occurs in T1DM.
   • Dehydration, stomach pain.
   • Nausea.
   • Fruity breath.
   • Drowsiness, vomiting.
   • Rapid breathing.
   • Headache.
   • Muscle pain.

8. • Cold or clammy skin.
   • Buzzing in ears.
   • Dizziness or lightheadedness.
   • Double or blurred vision.
   • Elevated heart rate.
   • Inability to do basic math.
   • Insomnia.
   • Irritability.
   • Confusion.
   • Paleness.
   • Shaking hands.

- Extreme fatigue.
- Headache.
- Nausea.
- Nervousness.
- Nightmares.
- Poor coordination.
- Restlessness.
- Slurred speech.
- Sweating.
- Visual spots.
- Extreme hunger; panicky hunger.
- Loss of consciousness.
- Seizures.
- Coma.

9. CVD, neuropathy and amputations, retinopathy and blindness, nephropathy, and dental disease.
10. Reduce risk of complications by 40%.

Chapter 3: Treatment of Diabetes

1. Physician, registered dietitian and/or certified diabetes educator, nurse, and exercise specialist.
2. To reduce significant fluctuations in blood glucose level.
3. High-fiber diet.
4. False (oral medications only used in type 2 diabetes, unless someone with type 1 DM becomes insulin resistant).
5. 70–120 mg/dl.
6. False.

Chapter 4: Exercise and Diabetes

1. Exercise increases glucose utilization, increases insulin sensitivity, and generally lowers blood glucose.
2. Their health history, including complications of diabetes, medication use, exercise goals, and what the likely glycemic response to exercise will be depending on type of exercise, nutrition surrounding exercise and level of insulization, blood glucose level prior to exercise and climate and stress.
3. • Lower blood sugar levels and improve the body's ability to use glucose.
   • Augment the blood glucose-lowering effect of injected insulin, therefore reducing the amount of insulin or hypoglycemic medication needed.

- Delay or prevent the development of atherosclerosis and risk factors related to heart disease, including blood pressure and elevated lipids, which are major threats to people with diabetes.
- Modify body composition and reduce weight when combined with a reduction in caloric intake. Weight loss and exercise increases insulin sensitivity and may allow those with diabetes to reduce the amount of insulin or oral hypoglycemic medication.
- Increase circulation to all parts of the body and therefore lessening the risk for the long-term complication of impaired circulation.
- Reduce depression, a common occurrence in those with diabetes.
- Reduce stress.
- Allow one with diabetes to live a 'normal life'. Some clients may be feel limited in exercise by their diabetes, however, you can educate them on how to safely engage in physical activity from walking to running to sports.

Hypoglycemia is low blood glucose, less than 70 mg/dl. The symptoms are:
- Abnormal gait
- Clicking feet when running
- Lack of balance
- Fatigue, "puniness"
- Confusion
- Seeing stars
- Chills
- Clammy
- Buzzing in ears
- Increased heart rate
- Shaky hands
- Irritability
- Reduction in power (cannot keep up with workout out partners, perform at usual level)
- Heart palpitations

To treat hypoglycemia eat 15 grams of carbohydrate (4 oz juice, 8 oz sports drink, ½ banana, 1 cup milk) and recheck blood glucose in 15 minutes.

4. See above answer
5. False
6. • Blood glucose level prior to exercise
   - Intensity, duration, and type of exercise
   - Level of circulating insulin (insulinization)
   - Food and fluid intake surrounding exercise
   - Climate and stress

7. a) increase, b) decrease, c) decrease but not as much as in longer-duration, lower-intensity exercise
8. The level of circulating insulin.
9. High.
10. • Level of insulinization surrounding exercise.
    • Pre-exercise meal.
    • Pre-exercise insulin adjustments.
    • During-exercise carbohydrate supplementation.
    • During-exercise hydration plan.
    • During-exercise insulin adjustments.
    • Postexercise carbohydrate supplementation.
    • Postexercise insulin adjustments.
11. True.
12. 100 mg/dl; 250 mg/dl with ketones or 350 mg/dl with or without ketones.
13. Insulinization is low; blood glucose levels will likely increase during exercise.
14. You suspect that his glucose levels are running high and you advise him to check his glucose levels immediately.
15. Decrease

Chapter 5: Exercise Design

1. At least 150 minutes per week of moderate-intensity aerobic physical activity. At least 2 times per week, on nonconsecutive days, of resistance training.
2. Proliferative diabetic retinopathy.
3. a. Leonora: cardiovascular exercise at light intensity, such as swimming, stationary cycling, or chair exercise (because she has peripheral neuropathy, walking may not be comfortable); also encourage lifestyle activities such as gardening or housework; light strength training once per week; starting with bouts of 10 minutes one time per week and increasing depending on her tolerance to exercise
   b. Jim: Moderate to vigorous intensity cardiovascular exercise and strength training; increase the duration or the frequency of exercise depending on tolerance to exercise.

Chapter 6: Nutrition Surrounding Exercise

1. Eat 15 grams of carbohydrate, recheck in 15 minutes and blood glucose should rise about 50 points.

2. A carbohydrate rich meal or snack with water before, water during, and a small snack that contains carbohydrate and water after.

3. Same as for the 30 minute run, but with 30-60 grams of carbohydrate during the ride.

Chapter 7: Special Considerations for Diabetes and Exercise

1. c. Check glucose before, during and after exercise; she is at increased risk for hypoglycemia; symptoms are: abnormal gait, clicking feet when running, lack of balance, fatigue, confusion, seeing stars, chills, clammy, buzzing in ears, increased heart rate, shaky hands, irritability, reduction in power (cannot keep up with workout out partners, perform at usual level), heart palpitations.

2. You may infer from her frustration that she is not meeting her blood glucose goals surrounding exercise; to motivate her emphasize the benefits of exercise and focus on consistency in her workouts (mode, intensity, duration, time of day etc); encourage her to keep a workout/blood glucose log and offer to review it with her.

3. Yes, it is safe because she tests her glucose level and is in glycemic control, she is otherwise healthy and her pregnancy is not complicated and she has been exercising regularly for the past year. The warning signs that exercise may increase risk to the mother or baby are: vaginal bleeding, leakage of amniotic fluid, preterm labor, decreased fetal movement, shortness of breath or labored breathing before exertion, headache, dizziness, muscle weakness, and calf pain or swelling.

4. Light cardiovascular exercise initially in short bouts of 5-10 minutes and increasing to 30 minutes 5 times per week, light to moderate strength training 1-2 times per week using light weights at 10-15 repetitions, incorporating balance work; because she has peripheral neuropathy, she may not be able to feel her pulse, use the talk test or the RPE scale to assess the intensity of her workout.

5. Increase carbohydrate intake (possibly adding sports drinks) during exercise and suggest that he discuss with his physician a further decrease in his basal rate reduction of insulin

Chapter 8: Professional responsibilities

1. • Stop, discontinue exercise, and check blood sugar if a meter is available.
   • Have the client ingest quick-acting CHO such as orange juice, Fig New-tons, non-diet soda or Lifesavers. Recheck blood sugar. If within normal ranges client may resume exercise when symptoms disappear.
   • Resume activity only when blood sugar levels are appropriate.
   • Client should ingest more substantial CHO in addition to some protein after exercise.
   • If the condition continues on a regular basis, refer the client to his/her physician.
2. • Too much food intake elevates blood sugar levels.
   • Too little insulin prevents enough glucose from entering the cells.
   • Illness, stress, infection may increase blood sugar.
3. • Consume adequate carbohydrate before and during exercise as indicted by the client's blood glucose before exercise and type/duration of exer-cise.
   • Consume a CHO snack following prolonged exercise.
   • Adjust insulin dosage accordingly.
   • Avoid injecting insulin into vigorously exercised muscle.
   • Carry quick-acting sugar during exercise.
   • Monitor blood sugar prior to, during, and after exercise.
   • Avoid starting exercise with blood glucose <100 mg/dl
4. • Excessive fatigue.
   • Signs or symptoms of hypoglycemia or hyperglycemia.
   • Abnormal muscle or joint discomfort or pain.
   • Inappropriate shortness of breath (SOB).
   • Dizziness, lightheadedness, nausea, confusion.
   • Excessive tachycardia or inappropriate bradycardia.
   • Leg pain, cramping.
   • Failure to increase HR with increased workload.
   • Onset of angina with exercise.
   • Client requests to stop the exercise.

✳ REFERENCES

Abate, N., and M. Chandalia. 2003. The impact of ethnicity on type 2 diabetes. *Journal of Diabetes Complications* 17:39–58.

American Academy of Clinical Endocrinologists Diabetes Mellitus Clinical Practice Guidelines Task Force. 2008. American Association of Clinical Endocrinologists medical guidelines for clinical practice for the management of diabetes mellitus. *Endocrine Practice* 13:Suppl 1.

American College of Sports Medicine (ACSM). 2007. Position stand: Exercise and fluid replacement. http://www.acsm-msse.org/pt/pt-core/template-journal/msse/media/0207.pdf

———. 2010. *Guidelines for exercise testing and prescription.* 8th ed. Philadelphia: Williams and Wilkins.

American College of Sports Medicine (ACSM) and American Diabetes Association. 2010. Exercise and type 2 diabetes: Joint position statement. *Medicine and Science in Sports and Exercise* 42 (12):2282–2303. http://journals.lww.com/acsm-msse/Fulltext/2010/12000/Exercise_and_Type_2_Diabetes__American_College_of.18.aspx (accessed March 31, 2011).

American Diabetes Association. 2002. Position statement: Diabetes mellitus and exercise. *Diabetes Care* 25:S64.

American Diabetes Association. 2008. Standards of medical care. *Diabetes Care* 31;1: S12.

American Dietetics Association (ADA) and American College of Sports Medicine (ACSM). 2000. Position of the American Dietetic Association, Dietitians of Canada, and American College of Sports Medicine: Nutrition and athletic performance. *Journal of the American Dietetics Association* 1001:543–1556.

American Heart Association. 2007. Resistance exercise in individuals with and without cardiovascular disease: 2007 update. http://www.americanheart.org/presenter.jhtml?identifier=3050002 accessed January 23, 2009.

———. 2009. ABCs of preventing heart disease, stroke, and heart attack. www.americanheart.org/presenter.jthml?identifier=3035374 accessed March 12, 2009.

Banerji, M. A., and H. E. Lebovitz. 1992. Insulin action in black Americans with NIDDM. *Diabetes Care* 15:1295–1302.

Bellenir, Karen, ed. 1999. *Diabetes sourcebook health reference series.* 2nd ed. Detroit: Omnigraphics.

Buse, J. B., N. H. Ginsberg, G. L. Bakris, N. G.Clark, F. Costa, V. Fonseca, H. C. Gerstein, S. Grundy, W. Nestor, M. P. Pignone, J. Plutzky, D. Porte, R. Redberg, K. F. Stitzel, and N. J. Stone. 2007. Primary prevention of cardiovascular disease in people with diabetes mellitus: A scientific statement from the American Heart Association and the American Diabetes Association. *Circulation* 115:114–126.

Casillas J. M., V. Gremeaux, S. Damake, A. Feki, and D. Pérennou. 2007. Exercise training for patients with cardiovascular disease. *Annales de Réadaptation et de Médecine Physique* 50:403–418.

References

Centers for Disease Control and Prevention (CDC). 2007. Diabetes fact sheet. http://www.cdc.gov/diabetes/pubs/factsheet07.htm (accessed November 24, 2008)

———. 2008a. Fast stats. http://www.cdc.gov/nchs/fastats/overwt.htm (accessed November 24, 2008)

———. 2008b. Prevalence of overweight and obesity among adults with diagnosed diabetes—United States, 1988–1994 and 1999–2002. MMRW Morb Mortal Wkly Rep. 2004;53:1066-1068. http://www.cdc.gov/mmwr/preview/mmwrhtml/mm5345a2.htm. (accessed November 24, 2008)

Ceysens, G., D. Rouiller, and M. Boulvain. 2006. Exercise for diabetic pregnant women. *Cochrane Database of Systematic Reviews* issue 3. Art. No.:CD004225.

Colberg, Sheri R. 2009. *Diabetic athlete's handbook.* Champaign, IL: Human Kinetics.

Diabetes Forecast. 2009. *Resource Guide.* Diabetes Forecast. January.

Dixon, L. B., J. Sundquist, and M. Winkleby. 2000. Differences in energy, nutrient, and food intakes in a U.S. sample of Mexica-America women and men: Findings from the Third National Health and Nutrition Examination Survey, 1988–1994. *American Journal of Epidemiology* 152:548–557.

Dornhorst, A., and M. Rossi. 1998. Risk and prevention of type 2 diabetes in women with gestational diabetes. *Diabetes Care* 21:B43–B49.

Franz, M. J., J. L. Boucher, J. Green-Pastors, and M. A. Powers. 2008. Evidence-based nutrition practice guidelines for diabetes and scope and standards of practice. *Journal of the American Dietetic Association* 108(4 Suppl 1):S52–8.

Gahagan, S., and J. Silverstein. 2003. Prevention and treatment of type 2 diabetes mellitus in children, with special emphasis on American Indian and Alaska Native children. American Academy of Pediatrics Committee on Native American Child Health. *Pediatrics* 112:e328.

Healthways. 2007. Impact of physical activity on specific chronic conditions. *Chronic Health Conditions, Exercise and the SilverSneakers Fitness Program.* Healthways SilverSneakers Fitness Program brochure. Franklin, TN: Healthways.

Healthways. 2008. *Group exercise instructor manual: Muscular strength and range of movement.* Franklin, TN: Healthways.

Kelly, C., and G. Booth. 2004. Diabetes in Canadian women. *BMC Women's Health* 4:S16–S24.

Kempf, K., W. Rathmann, and H. Christian. 2008. Impaired glucose regulation and type 2 diabetes in children and adolescents. *Diabetes Metabolism Research and Reviews* 24:427–437.

Lee, B. L. 2003. Racial differences in diabetes mellitus. *International Journal of Opthamology* 43:39–46.

Lisle, D. K., and T. H.Trojian. 2006. Managing the athlete with type 1 diabetes. *Current Sports Medicine Reports* 5:93–98.

Liu, S., J. E. Manson, and M. J. Stampfer. 2000. A prospective study of whole-grain intake and risk of type 2 diabetes mellitus in U.S. women. *American Journal of Public Health* 90:1409–1415.

Mattola, M. 2008. The role of exercise in the prevention and treatment of gestational diabetes mellitus. *Current Sports Medicine Reports* 6:381–386.

Narayan, K. M., J. P. Boyle, T. J. Thompson, S. W. Sorensen, and D. F. Williamson. 2003. Lifetime risk for diabetes mellitus in the United States. *Journal of the American Medical Association* 290:1884–1890.

National Institute of Diabetes, Digestive and Kidney Diseases (NIDDK). 2001. Diet and exercise dramatically delay type 2 diabetes: Diabetes medication Metformin also effective. http://www2.niddk.nih.gov/News/SearchNews/08_08_2001.htm (accessed April 24, 2009).

———. 2009. National diabetes clearinghouse. http://diabetes.niddk.nih.gov/dm/pubs/statistics/ (accessed January 4, 2009).

National Institutes of Health. 2005. National diabetes fact sheet: United States 2005. www.ndep.nih.gov/diabetes/pubs/2005_National_Diabetes_Fact_Sheet.pdf. (accessed November 25, 2008).

Nelson, M., W. Rejeski, S. Blair, P. Duncan, J. Judge, A. King, C. Macera, and C. Castaneda-Sceppa. 2007. Physical activity and public health in older adults: Recommendation from the American College of Sports Medicine and the American Heart Association [Special communications: Special reports]. *Medicine & Science in Sports and Exercise* 9(8):1435–1445.

Neufeld, N. D., L. J. Raffel, C. Landon, Y. D. Chen, and C. M. Vadheim. 1998. Early presentation of type 2 diabetes in Mexican-American youth. *Diabetes Care* 21:80–86.

Nguyen, H. G., M. L. Maciejewski, S. Gao, E. Lin, B. Williams, and J. P. LoGerfo. 2008. Health care use and costs associated with use of a health club membership benefit in older adults with diabetes. *Diabetes Care* 31: 1562–1567.

Pedersen, B. K., and B. Saltin. 2006. Evidence for prescribing exercise as therapy in chronic disease. *Scandinavian Journal of Medicine and Science in Sports* 16(Supp 1): 3–63.

Sigal, R. J., G. P. Kenny, D. H. Wasserman, C. Castane da-Sceppa, and R. D. White. 2006. Physical activity/exercise and type 2 diabetes: A consensus statement from the American Diabetes Association. *Diabetes Care* 29, 6:1433–1438.

Tuomilheto, J., J. Lindstom, and J. G. Eriksson, T. T. Valle, H. Hamalainen, P. Ilanne-Parikka, Keinanen-Kiukaanniemis, M. Laakso, A. Louheranta, M. Rastas, V. Salminen, and A. Uusitupa. 2001. Prevention of type 2 diabetes mellitus by changes in lifestyle among subjects with impaired glucose tolerance. *New England Journal of Medicine* 344:1343–1350.

United States Department of Health and Human Services (HHS). 2009. Physical activity guidelines for adults. www.health.gov/paguidelines (accessed January 23, 2009).

Wallberg-Henriksson, H. 1992. Exercise and diabetes mellitus. *Exercise and Sport Science Review* 20.

The Writing Group for the SEARCH for Diabetes in Youth Study Group. 2007. Incidence of diabetes in youth in the United States. *Journal of the American Medical Association* 297:2716–2724.

Zhang C., C. Solomon, J. Manson, and F. B. Hu. 2006. A prospective study of progravid physical activity and sedentary behaviors in relation to the risk for gestational diabetes mellitus. *Archives of Internal Medicine* 166:543–548.

✳ | RESOURCES

ASSOCIATIONS/ORGANIZATIONS

American College of Sports Medicine (ACSM)
401 W Michigan St
Indianapolis, IN 46202
(317) 637-9200
Fax: (317) 634-7817
www.ACSM.org

American Diabetes Association
1660 Duke Street
Alexandria, VA 22314
1-800-232-3472 or (703) 549-1550
www.diabetes.org

Canadian Diabetes Association
15 Toronto St, Ste 800
Toronto, ON M5C 2E3 Canada
1-800-BANTING or (416) 363-3373
E-mail: info@cola-nat.org
www.diabetes.ca

International Diabetes Center
5000 W 39th St.
Minneapolis MN 55416
612-927-3393
www.idcdiabetes.com

International Diabetic Athletes Association
1647-B West Bethany Home Road
Phoenix, AZ 85015
1-800-898-IDAA or (602) 433-2113
Fax: (602) 433-9331
E-mail: idaa@diabetes-exercise.org
www.diabetes-exercise.org

National Diabetes Education Program (NDEP)
NIDDK, National Institutes of Health
Bethesda, MD 20892
1-800-438-5383
www.ndep.nih.gov

BOOKS

American College of Sports Medicine (ACSM). *ACSM's Resource Manual for Guidelines for Exercise Testing and Prescription.* 8th ed. Baltimore: Lippincott Williams & Wilkins, 2010.

Colberg, Sheri R. *Diabetic Athlete's Handbook.* Champaign, IL: Human Kinetics, 2009.

✳ ABOUT THE AUTHORS

Hana Abdulaziz Feeney, MS, RD, CSSD, a native Tucsonan, is the owner of Nourishing Results, an integrative nutrition private practice. She completed her bachelor's of science in exercise science at Arizona State University and earned her master's of science in nutritional sciences at the University of Arizona. She is a registered dietitian and a board certified specialist in sports dietetics. As a nutrition coach, Hana empowers individuals through continuous support to create positive behavior changes and achieve optimal health through conscious eating and physical activity. It is her mission to provide education and tools that inspire each individual to find his or her way to fulfilled living. Hana specializes is weight management, type 1 and type 2 diabetes, sports nutrition, autoimmunity, digestive health, cardiovascular disease, and inflammatory disorders. She lectures regularly in the community on a variety of topics, continually develops new educational materials, leads a weekly Nutrition and Exercise Performance workshop, and holds a weekly radio segment. As a nutritionist at a health resort, she provides one-on-one consultations on topics ranging from prevention and treatment of chronic disease to optimizing body composition and nutritional supplementation.

Gwen Hyatt, MS, founded DSWFitness (Desert Southwest Fitness, Inc.) in 1980 to provide continuing education for fitness, health, rehabilitation and clinical professionals. With a double master's degree in exercise science and gerontology, Gwen is highly respected for her work with exercise in aging and special populations. She has authored 14 correspondence courses and presented at more than 20 IDEA conventions. Students in 50 states and 48 countries have registered for courses published by DSWFitness.

Gwen is a former faculty member at Bemidji State University and the University of Arizona. She has been the recipient of the 2005 ACE Fitness Educator of the Year Award, the Southern Arizona Small Business Award for Excellence as a Woman-Owned Business, the Utah Fitness Instructors Association Leadership Award and the Arthur Anderson Small Business Award.

To celebrate turning 50, Gwen participated in her first century cycling event and has since completed eleven centuries and six half plus centuries, placing platinum in her last event. At the age of 55, Gwen decided to jump into multisport competitions and completed her first triathlon. In the past year she has competed in six triathlons, finishing no lower than second place in her age group.

For over twenty-five years, Gwen has been an industry educator and role model and has served the industry with integrity, professionalism and passion.